# GET OUT!

## A shrink's guide to using the great outdoors as therapy

Dr. Patricia A. Farrell

Book cover photo: Patty Brito on Unsplash.com

Amazon author page for P. A. Farrell: https://tinyurl.com/4zk9pfe6 AND https://tinyurl.com/t8xkp4zx

**The Pocket Companion Series contains:**

*When Your Mind Won't Stop*

*After the Loss: Finding Your Way Through Grief*

*You Are Enough: Rebuilding Your Self-Worth*

*At the Crossroads: Making Decisions When Nothing Feels Clear*

*When People Hurt: Navigating Difficult Relationships*

*When You Feel Stuck: Finding Movement in Hard Times*

**Books by Patricia A. Farrell, Ph.D.**

When You Can't Pour From an Empty Glass: CBT Skills for Exhausted Caregivers

The Little Book on Learning Big Critical Thinking Skills

The Smart Kid's Survival Guide: Making Good Choices in a Confusing World

How to Be Your Own Therapist

It's Not All in Your Head: Anxiety, Depression, Mood Swings and Multiple Sclerosis

Unfiltered: Beneath the noise of our thoughts lies the true narrative of our minds

Unfiltered Again: A behind-the-scenes look at healthcare, medicine and mental health

A Social Security Disability Psychological Claims Handbook: A simple guide to understanding your SSD claim for psychological impairments and unraveling the maze of decision-making

A Social Security Disability Psychological Claims Guidebook for Children's Benefits

The Disability Accessible US Parks in All 50 States: A Comprehensive Guide

Birding in the US NOW!: A birding guide for individuals with disabilities

# Contents

# Introduction: The Thing That Was There All Along

I want to start with a question, and I want you to actually think about it before you continue reading.

When was the last time you felt genuinely, honestly good? *Not "fine." Not "managing." Not "could be worse."* Actually good—the kind of good where your body feels like it belongs to you again, your mind stops spinning, and you get this quiet sense that whatever is coming next, you can handle it. Do you know what I mean?

Got it? Good. Now, where were you?

I have asked some version of that question to hundreds of people over the years. And the answers land in the same place with almost eerie consistency. A walk on the beach. A morning on the porch before anyone else was awake. A road trip where you pulled over just to look at something—a mountain, a river, a field going gold in late afternoon light. A thunderstorm you stopped to actually watch instead of grumbling about.

These are the types of memories people also use when they want to fall asleep at night because they felt so good being in that place, or looking at that river, mountain, or whatever. That way you can relax and go to sleep.

Outside. The answer is almost always outside.

You probably weren't thinking of it as therapy at the time. You were just... there. And something in you settled in a way it hadn't all week. Maybe all month.

This book is about that settling. What it actually is. Why it happens. And—here's the part most people miss—how to stop waiting for it to happen by accident.

## The Answer Nobody Wanted to Fund

**Here's something that should probably make you a bit angry.**

For decades, researchers at universities and medical centers around the world have been quietly publishing study after study showing that spending time outside does extraordinary things to the human brain and body. Stress hormones drop. Blood pressure falls. The part of the brain linked to depression and anxious overthinking goes quiet. The immune system gets a measurable boost. Sleep improves. Attention sharpens. Mood lifts—not in a vague "I feel a little better" way, but in ways you can measure with blood tests and brain scans. It's real and not imaginary.

These effects show up in children and elderly people. In people with serious depression and people who thought they were doing fine. In rainy countries and sunny ones. Across cultures and continents. And they start showing up in as little as twenty to thirty minutes. That's pretty quick, isn't it?

Twenty to thirty minutes. Sitting. Walking slowly. Just being outside.

And yet most people have never heard any of this. It wasn't on the evening news. It didn't trend online. It didn't make its way into doctors' offices or mental health clinics in any meaningful way. We didn't even see the "influencers" shouting about it online. If they weren't promoting it, what was happening?

Why not? Here's the uncomfortable answer: there is no money in it. No pharmaceutical company profits when you take a walk in the park. No device to sell. No subscription to charge. Treatments that are free and available to almost everyone don't attract the kind of funding that gets turned into TV commercials and clinical guidelines. So, the research sat in journals, and the rest of us kept filling prescriptions and booking therapy appointments and wondering why something was still missing.

To be very clear: therapy and medication are real, valuable tools and I've used both in my practice. But they work best when they're not the only tool in the box. And for most people, the outdoors is a tool that's been sitting untouched for years.

## Full Disclosure: I Used to Hate This Idea

Before we go any further, I owe you some honesty.

I am not a naturally outdoorsy person. I grew up in a major world city. My idea of a perfect Saturday involved the library, not a trailhead. I did not own hiking boots and had no particular interest in changing that. When friends suggested camping, I became mysteriously unavailable. When coworkers talked about weekend hikes, I nodded politely and prayed they wouldn't invite me. I couldn't understand how anybody could sleep in a tent and not worry about wild animals or terrible insects.

I was also, for many of those years, quietly running on fumes. Long hours. Heavy caseloads. The specific exhaustion that comes from spending your days fully present for other people's hardest moments. I was good at my job. I was not good at refilling myself from what that job was taking from me.

About fifteen years ago, I stumbled into the research on nature and mental health. I wasn't looking for it—it kept showing up in the scientific journals I was reading, insistently, like a neighbor who won't stop knocking. And because I'm someone who follows evidence even when it inconveniences me, I made myself pay attention.

Then, reluctantly, I made myself go outside.

I started with five minutes. Literally five minutes on a park bench during my lunch break, phone in my pocket, timer set so I'd know when I was allowed to go back inside. I felt slightly ridiculous. I also felt restless and impatient and fairly certain I was wasting time I could spend being productive.

And then, gradually, something shifted.

The mental noise got quieter. The feeling of running perpetually behind started to ease up. I began sleeping through the night. People told me I seemed like a calmer version of myself. Nothing in my actual life had changed—same job, same pressures, same stack of unread emails. But I was handling all of it differently.

The only thing I had added was thirty minutes outside every day. That was it.

I tell you this not to sell you on a lifestyle but to let you know that I've stood exactly where you might be standing right now—skeptical, busy, not especially drawn to nature, and pretty sure this doesn't apply to you. It applied to me. It likely applies to you.

## What This Book Actually Is

Let me be straight with you about what you've picked up.

This is not a hiking book. It is not a camping book. It will not ask you to forage for berries, identify trees, or invest in gear. There is no chapter about waking up at dawn to watch the sunrise (unless you want there to be, and if so, Chapter 4 will make you glad you did).

This is a book about what happens inside you when you go outside. The actual biology. The actual psychology. The research that most people will never see because it lives in academic journals behind paywalls, written in the kind of language that was specifically designed to be unreadable by anyone who didn't go to graduate school.

I went to graduate school. I read the journals. And then I translated them into something useful.

Each chapter takes one piece of the outdoor experience and pulls it apart—what the science says, why it matters, and what to actually do with that information. Here's the roadmap:

Chapter 1 lays the foundation—what is genuinely happening in your brain and nervous system the moment you step outside. Once you understand this, everything else makes sense in a whole new way.

Chapter 2 is about your nose, which turns out to be doing a lot more than you thought. The compounds released by trees. The chemistry of petrichor—that smell after rain. The way outdoor scents signal your nervous system to relax. Strange but true, and the research is fascinating.

Chapter 3 is about water. Seeing it. Hearing it. Being near it. Scientists call it the "blue mind" effect, and once you read the evidence, you will never stand at the edge of a lake or an ocean the same way again.

Chapter 4 is about sunlight—not as a skincare concern, but as one of the most powerful biological regulators your brain has. Mood. Sleep. Energy. Immune function. All of it tied to something that's literally free and available every single day.

Chapter 5 looks at movement in nature and why the same walk produces different results outdoors versus on a treadmill. (The treadmill people are not going to love this chapter.)

Chapter 6 is about sound—specifically, what the constant noise of modern life is doing to your stress response, and what happens when you replace it with the sounds your ears were actually built to process.

Chapter 7 addresses loneliness, which is quietly doing more damage to public health than almost anyone wants to talk about, and the surprising role that outdoor time plays in interrupting it.

Chapter 8 is where we get honest about the obstacles. Bad weather, no time, physical limitations, safety concerns, living somewhere that doesn't look anything like a nature documentary. These are real barriers and they deserve real answers.

Chapter 9 is the one nobody wants to read but everybody needs: how to actually make this a habit. Because knowing something is good for you has never once been enough to guarantee you'll do it, and we both know it. About it how much exercise equipment have you bought and never used? Think about all the New Year's resolutions about getting in shape and losing weight that were never kept.

Chapter 10, the final chapter, is about the long game. What a life with regular outdoor time actually looks like—and what you stand to gain by starting now rather than later.

## A Few Things to Know Before We Start

This book is not a substitute for professional mental health treatment. If you are dealing with serious depression, anxiety, trauma, or any condition that a physician or therapist is helping you manage, keep going. Don't change your medication. Don't quit therapy. What I'm offering here is something you add, not something you swap.

Also, you don't need to live near anything impressive. The research is remarkably consistent on this point—you don't need wilderness. You don't need a national park or a pristine lake or any of the scenery you see on nature calendars. A neighborhood park counts. A tree-lined block counts. A patch of sky visible from your fire escape counts. Studies done in dense urban areas show many of the same benefits as studies done in forests. Start with what you have. Where you are.

And you don't need to feel it working for it to work. Your cortisol (the stress hormone) doesn't wait for you to feel relaxed before it starts dropping. Your nervous system doesn't require your buy-in. The biology operates on its own schedule, whether you believe in it or not. That actually makes this easier: you don't have to try very hard. You mostly just have to show up. Showing up, that's the ticket.

## The Objection I Know You're Already Forming

Somewhere in the back of your mind, a voice is saying: this is too simple.

I know that voice. I had it too. We have all been trained to believe that real medicine is complicated, that genuine healing requires intensive effort and expensive expertise, and that anything this accessible and this free can't possibly be serious science.

But think about it for a second. Sleep is simple. Drinking water is simple. Eating food rather than not eating food is simple. Nobody questions those things. Nobody calls them "*alternative medicine*."

The most fundamental things that keep human beings functioning tend to be the least complicated—and the ones we most consistently skip because they don't feel like they should be enough.

Here is the thing about going outside: your brain evolved outdoors. Every single one of your ancestors, going back hundreds of thousands of years, lived their entire life under the sky. The nervous system you were born with was shaped by sunlight and wind and moving water and the sound of leaves. Those aren't decorative details. Those are the operating conditions your brain was built for.

Today, most of us spend over ninety percent of our time indoors. And we're genuinely puzzled about why we feel so out of it.

Going outside isn't a wellness trend. It's not an alternative therapy or a lifestyle choice. It's giving your brain and body back the one thing they were literally designed to run on.

Okay. Let's Go.

My invitation to you is simple: read the chapters that follow, understand why this works, and then try it—actually try it, consistently, for a few weeks. Not dramatically. Not by transforming yourself into someone who posts sunrise hikes on social media. Just outside, regularly, paying attention to what happens.

Not what you expect to happen. Not what I'm promising will happen. What actually happens, in your body and your mood and your ability to get through a difficult Tuesday.

I think you're going to be surprised. I was.

The thing that was there all along—right outside your door, free, available every single day—has been waiting for you to notice it.

**Time to go find out what it can do.**

# Chapter 1: Why Going Outside Actually Works

Here is something that might surprise you about this book: it was written by someone who used to dislike being outside.

Not just dislike it. Actually, I hated it. Give me a climate-controlled office, a comfortable chair, and a good book any day. The outdoors? That was for other people. People who owned hiking boots and knew how to identify birds. People who seemed to have some secret manual for enjoying nature that I had never received.

I grew up in a major city. My childhood weekends were spent at the library, not at parks. My idea of a good time was reading in my bedroom, not climbing trees or exploring trails. When friends suggested camping trips, I'd make excuses. When coworkers talked about weekend hikes, I'd change the subject.

Nature wasn't for me. Or so I thought.

Then about fifteen years ago, I hit a wall. I was working long hours as a psychologist, and I started noticing something that bothered me. The techniques I had learned in graduate school—the ones that were supposed to help people with depression and anxiety—were working, sure. But they felt incomplete. Like I was handing people tools without showing them where to use those tools.

That's when I started digging into the research on outdoor time and mental health. And what I found changed everything about how I think about well-being.

## The Science Nobody Talks About

Here's what most people don't know: there are thousands of scientific studies on how being outside affects our brains and bodies. Not New Age ideas. Not wellness trends. Actual peer-reviewed research from major universities and medical centers around the world.

And the results are staggering.

Studies show that spending time in nature *reduces cortisol*—that's your body's main stress hormone. *It lowers blood pressure. It improves immune function. It reduces inflammation throughout your body.* These aren't small effects. We're talking about changes you can measure in blood tests.

But it goes deeper than that. Being outside changes what's happening in your brain. It affects the parts of your brain responsible for rumination—that endless loop of negative thoughts that keeps you up at night. It impacts the areas involved in emotional regulation. It even changes patterns of brain activity associated with depression.

One study out of Stanford University took people for a ninety-minute walk. Half walked through a natural area with trees and grass. Half walked through an urban environment with buildings and traffic. Afterward, researchers used brain imaging to look at what was happening in their brains.

The people who walked in nature showed decreased activity in the part of the brain *associated with rumination and depression*—the subgenual prefrontal cortex. This is the area that lights up when you're stuck in negative thought patterns.

The urban walkers? *No change.* Same brain activity before and after. You must be asking yourself right now, "How could there have been this kind of difference when they were both just walking?" It wasn't the walking, but where they were walking made all the difference.

Ninety minutes. One walk. Measurable changes in brain activity. How simple is that?

Another study from the University of Michigan found that people who spent just twenty to thirty minutes in a natural setting showed *significant reductions in cortisol levels.* Pretty much we've all had some association with cortisol and it's *always been a negative one* because this is the *stress hormone.* Researchers here called that a natural setting a "*nature pill.*" They weren't asking people to hike or exercise or do anything strenuous. Just sit or walk slowly in a natural environment—no phones, no work, just being there. The effects showed up in **less than half an hour**.

When I first read these studies, I remember thinking, if we could bottle this and sell it as a drug, it would be the biggest pharmaceutical breakthrough in decades. But we can't bottle it. Because it's not a chemical. *It's an experience.* It's what happens when you take your brain and body—which evolved outdoors over hundreds of thousands of years—and put them back in the environment they were designed for.

Think about that for a moment. Your brain evolved in nature. Every ancestor you have, going back hundreds of thousands of years, lived outside. They spent their entire lives surrounded by trees, water, animals, and weather. They never saw a building. Never looked at a screen. Never sat under artificial light.

And now? Most of us spend over *ninety percent of our time indoors.* That's really an excessive amount of time to spend indoors. We wake up in a building, drive to another building, sit there all day, and drive home. Maybe we step outside to walk to our car or check the mail. That's a massive disconnect. And our brains and bodies are suffering because of it.

## Your Brain on Nature

Your brain is constantly processing information: sights, sounds, sensations, thoughts. In a typical indoor environment—home, office, or car—your brain operates in what researchers call "*directed attention.*" You're focusing on specific things. Reading emails. Watching TV. Scrolling through your phone. Directed attention takes effort. It requires you to actively block out distractions and force your focus onto whatever you're doing. It's like holding a heavy weight—you can do it for a while, but eventually your muscles give out.

This is why you feel exhausted after a day of work even if you never left your desk. Your attention system is tired. Depleted. Used up. One thing I noticed about people who decided that, after a hard day's work in the office, they would go and play racquetball: I used to wonder where they got the energy to do that after a workday. I was naive. I didn't realize that playing that sport gave them a renewed sense of energy and well-being that counteracted all the sitting they did during the day.

They were exercising, but when you go outside in a natural environment, something different happens. Your attention shifts into what researchers call "*soft fascination.*" You notice things—a bird flying by, leaves moving in the wind, clouds drifting, water flowing—but you don't have to concentrate on them. Your attention is engaged but not effortful. It's the difference between studying for an exam and watching a beautiful sunset. Both engage your attention. But one drains you and the other restores you.

This gives the directed attention system a chance to rest and recharge. It's like letting an overworked muscle recover.

The researcher who identified this process, Rachel Kaplan at the University of Michigan, calls it *Attention Restoration Theory*. She found that natural environments have four key qualities that restore attention. **First**, they take you away from your usual demands and distractions. **Second,** they hold your attention effortlessly—nature is full of things that catch your eye without requiring hard focus. **Third**, they're rich and varied enough to keep you engaged without overwhelming you. And **fourth**, they align with what humans naturally find interesting and meaningful. We're drawn to nature because our brains evolved to pay attention to it. It feels right in a way that artificial environments don't.

This restoration isn't just about feeling less tired. Studies show that after spending time in nature, people *perform better on tests* requiring focused attention, make fewer mistakes, concentrate for longer periods, and show improved working memory. All of that happens to you, almost miraculously, without your doing a thing.

## Your Body's Stress Response

Being outside also affects something called your *autonomic nervous system*—the part that controls things you don't consciously direct: *heart rate, breathing, digestion, and the stress response.* "Autonomic" happens without any conscious effort. It's like a machine that keeps going and you don't have to turn a switch to get it to keep going. I think the only time we're conscious of breathing is when we have an allergy attack, asthma, or the common cold.

Your autonomic nervous system has *two main branches*. Think of them as *the gas pedal* and *the brake pedal* in a car. Simple enough, right? The *sympathetic* branch is your *gas pedal*—is the *"fight or flight" system*. It activates when you're stressed or threatened. Your heart rate goes up. Your breathing gets shallow. Your muscles tense. Your body prepares to deal with danger. I've always found that having some way to connect a system with a phrase or word is helpful in remembering it. For me, if I wanted to remember the sympathetic branch, I would think of someone saying to me, "**Step on it!**" So, it's the "go" part of the system.

The *parasympathetic* branch is your *brake pedal*—the *"rest and digest" system*. It activates when you're safe and relaxed. Your heart rate slows. Your breathing deepens. Your muscles release. Your body focuses on healing and recovery. If you want something to remember this, consider it being the "*pause*" instead of the break pedal.

In modern life, most of us spend too much time with the **gas pedal floored**. Traffic. Deadlines. Financial stress. Bad news. Your body doesn't know the difference between running from a predator and running late for a meeting. The stress response activates either way. And when the gas pedal is always pressed, *you burn* out, and burnout carries with it more negative effects than we want to think about. Your mood suffers. Sleep gets worse. You feel constantly on edge.

Being in nature *activates your brake pedal.* It shifts the balance from sympathetic to parasympathetic. Your body gets the message: *you're safe. You can relax. You can heal.* Healing is a part of this experience, as you will soon learn here.

One study measured heart rate variability in people *walking through different environments.* Higher heart rate variability means *your body can adapt flexibly*—speeding up when needed, slowing down when it's time to rest. People walking through forests showed significantly higher heart rate variability than people walking through urban areas. The forest walkers' bodies were operating in rest-and-digest mode. The urban walkers were still in fight-or-flight mode, even though they were just walking. In fact, they had brought the urban environment with all of its constant demands with them. Consider how *high a price we pay* in terms of our health, both physical and mental, because of urban environments and their consistent demands of us.

Another study showed participants either images of natural scenes or images of urban scenes while measuring heart rate and blood pressure. The people looking at nature images showed measurably lower heart rate and blood pressure within minutes. Just looking at pictures of trees and water was enough to activate the parasympathetic system. Looking at urban scenes produced no change at all.

Your body recognizes that being in nature is different from being in a building or a car—even when your conscious mind hasn't registered it. And it responds accordingly.

## The Biophilia Hypothesis

There's a term in psychology for this connection between humans and nature: *biophilia*. The word literally means *"love of life" or "love of living things."* The biophilia hypothesis, proposed by biologist E.O. Wilson, suggests that humans have an innate tendency to seek connections with nature and other forms of life. It might account for our love of cats and dogs.

This isn't just a philosophical idea. It makes evolutionary sense. For most of human history—about 300,000 years—humans lived outside. Not in houses. Not in cities. Outside. In forests, on grasslands, and near water sources. Our brains and bodies evolved in those environments. Everything about how we're wired was shaped by those years of living in nature. Of course, before Homo sapiens, there was a different form of human life, and they lived two million years ago.

Then, very recently in the grand sweep of human history, we started living in permanent structures. More recently still, we started living in cities. And in just the last few decades, we started spending most of our time indoors looking at screens. Our brains haven't caught up. We're still running internal brain software designed for the natural world, but we're trying to use it in buildings and vehicles.

That mismatch causes problems. Anxiety. Depression. Attention difficulties. Sleep disruption. A constant sense of being off, disconnected, like something is missing but you can't name it. Going outside addresses that fundamental mismatch. It gives your brain and body a chance to operate in the environment they were designed for. And that creates space for healing.

## But I Don't Live Near Nature

Here's what the research shows: *you don't need pristine wilderness.* You don't need untouched forest or remote mountains. You don't even need what most people think of as "real" nature. A small caveat here: you do need natural things, *not fake plants.* They won't do it. Do you know what will? Pictures of bucolic scenes of the ocean or of meadows and forests. That's pretty perplexing, isn't it? It just goes to show you that there are still wonders in the brain for us to discover and this is one of the contradictions.

Studies show that even small amounts of urban nature—city parks, tree-lined streets, and community gardens—provide significant mental health benefits. Quite a few decades ago, New York City realized the value of parks, even if they were tiny. Of course, this was the time when the urban environmentalist *Jane Jacobs* was holding sway and could point out to city managers the benefits of these small features and *Robert Moses* was fighting her to make everything concrete. He was instrumental in the building of the Cross Bronx Expressway and the construction of low-cost housing projects in New York City. In the process, he destroyed neighborhoods.

But, in contrast to what Robert Moses envisioned for this great city, others had a different view of what the city needed. They began to construct what were called "*pocket or vest-pocket parks*," small areas where people could go and sit among a few trees and bushes, with fixed benches along the side walls of the parks. They were no bigger than the size of one of the small brownstone homes that once stood there.

Research from the UK found that people living near even modest green spaces reported better mental health than those without nearby greenery. Another study concluded that office workers who could see trees from their window had lower stress levels than those with views of buildings. *Just seeing nature through a window made a measurable difference.* I remember having an office in a small, three-story building where, looking down from the third floor into a green space, I could see a lovely fruit tree, and it was enlivening. The office was really an enjoyable place to be and I never minded climbing up and down those steps multiple times a day.

You work with what you have. If there's a park within walking distance, that's your nature. A tree-lined street is your nature. A courtyard with some plants. A balcony where you can see the sky. Any rooftop where you can watch clouds and hear birds. The research is consistent: **something is always better than nothing**, and *many of the documented benefits show up in urban settings, not just wilderness areas.*

Is a city park as powerful as a dense forest? Probably not. After all, it wouldn't have those wonderful oils and scents that all of the forest trees float into the air. The research suggests that *more natural environments produce stronger effects.* But meaningful benefits occur across a wide range of outdoor contexts. The key isn't finding perfect nature. It's finding whatever nature is available to you and spending time there consistently. Start where you are. Use what you have. Do what you can.

## Why Most People Don't Go Outside

If being outside is this beneficial, why don't more people do it? There are a few honest reasons worth acknowledging.

**First,** we've been conditioned to *see outdoor time as optional*—as recreation, as something you do when you have extra time, not something essential to well-being. You wouldn't skip sleep for a week and expect to function normally. But we skip outdoor time without a second thought.

**Second**, modern life actively *discourages going outside.* Our jobs keep us indoors. Our entertainment is indoors. Our social lives happen indoors or online. Going outside requires a deliberate decision. Staying inside is frictionless.

**Third**, there's a cultural story that *outdoor life is for a certain type of person*. Athletic people. Outdoorsy people. People with gear and knowledge and the right clothes. But that belief doesn't hold up. You don't need special equipment to sit on a park bench. You don't need to identify birds to benefit from hearing them. You simply need to be outside.

**And fourth**—perhaps most importantly—many of us have *forgotten how to be somewhere without a clear purpose or goal.* The idea of sitting under a tree and doing nothing feels wasteful. Like laziness with better lighting. Being there can make us feel guilty and fidgety.

It's not laziness. It's maintenance. Understanding the difference is what this book is designed to help you do.

## My Own Journey

I want to be clear about where I'm coming from, because I'm not a naturally outdoorsy person. I am someone who had to learn this the hard way, and who resisted it for longer than made any sense.

When I first started making myself spend time outside, I was genuinely bad at it. I'd go to a park, sit on a bench, and within five minutes I'd be checking my phone. I couldn't just sit there. It felt uncomfortable. Boring. Like I was wasting time I should be spending being productive. Can you say "*constantly multitasking*"? If there's one thing that I think we need to tackle, it's multitasking and how it is, according to the research I've seen, an impossibility.

During the day, my mind would race through everything waiting for me—emails piling up, the laundry, calls I needed to return. I'd start mentally drafting to-do lists. Planning the week. Rehashing old conversations, things I should have done.

After several weeks, I began to realize that this restlessness was exactly the reason I needed to be outside. I had become so accustomed to constant motion and productivity that my brain had lost the ability to *simply be.* That's not a personality quirk. That's a symptom.

I started very small. Five minutes on my lunch break. I'd leave my office, walk to a nearby park, sit for exactly five minutes, and leave. I set a timer. I kept my phone in my pocket.

Those first five minutes felt like a long time. But gradually, something shifted. The mental chatter didn't disappear, but it softened. It became less urgent. More like background noise than a blaring alarm.

After a few weeks of five-minute breaks, I extended to ten minutes. Then fifteen. I started going in the morning before work. Then I added a weekend walk. Nothing strenuous. Just outside, slow and present. At one job in a suburban hospital, a friend and I would get into my car with our lunch and park at the edge of a field bordered with trees. A small herd of deer would come to feed. It was incredible. We sat there for our whole lunch hour, watching the deer, which would occasionally look up at us and then go back to grazing. The windows were open, and the breeze came in, the grass swayed back and forth. It was wonderful. But how many people have that luxury? At the time, we didn't even think about how lucky we were, but looking back now, I miss those lunch hours in the car near that meadow.

I never worked near a meadow again, but in a dense urban city, I managed to get out and walk for for almost a mile on my lunch hour. It felt good just being outside even if there were lots of people and cars.

Once I began to truly bring the outdoors into my life, the change was gradual, but it was real. I started feeling more resilient. Less rattled by daily stressors. More able to focus during work. Sleeping better. People noticed before I did. "You seem calmer," one of them said one evening. "Less on edge. What changed?"

The only thing that had changed was thirty minutes or so outside every day. Same job. Same pressures. Same responsibilities. But I was managing all of it better. That wasn't a coincidence. That was biology doing exactly what the research said it would do.

I'm telling you this because I want you to know that I understand the skepticism. I understand the voice that says this is too simple, or that it won't work for you, or that you don't have time. I had every one of those thoughts. ***And I was wrong about all of them.***

## What This Book Will Teach You

In the chapters that follow, I'm going to walk you through how to use the outdoors as a genuine tool for mental health—not as a replacement for professional care, but as a powerful and well-supported complement to it.

We'll cover the specific ways different outdoor environments affect your brain and body. Not all nature is the same. Forests affect you differently than open fields. Water has its own distinct benefits. The time of day matters. The season matters. The scents in the air matter. Each chapter takes one of these elements and *examines what the research actually shows.* These studies are the part that can help you clear up any concerns about using the environment effectively for your health.

We'll talk about how to get started if you've never thought of yourself as an outdoor person, or if you have physical limitations that make some activities difficult. The barriers are real, and we'll address them directly—bad weather, limited time, safety concerns, living in dense urban areas, and the simple resistance that comes from changing any long-standing habit.

Most importantly, we'll focus on sustainability—because one remarkable hike or a week-long nature retreat, while valuable, is not what the research recommends. The evidence consistently points toward *small, regular doses of outdoor time* as the most effective approach. Twenty minutes outside every day produces more lasting benefit than occasional larger experiences. Consistency matters more than intensity.

## What You Need to Know Before We Start

This book *isn't a substitute for professional mental health treatment,* as I've mentioned. If you're dealing with severe depression, anxiety, trauma, or any serious mental health condition, please work with a qualified professional. If you are on medication, *don't stop taking it.* If you are in therapy, keep going. If you are in crisis, please contact a crisis line or emergency services.

What I'm offering here is a *complementary approach*—something that works alongside professional care and that the research supports as genuinely useful. *It's not instead of anything.* It's in addition to it.

The most useful approach is curiosity rather than expectation. You're not trying to produce a specific outcome. You're experimenting with spending more time outside and paying attention to what happens in your body, your mood, your sleep, and your ability to cope with daily stress. *The data you gather from your own experience is the most relevant data you have.*

## One Last Thing

Before we move on, I want to address the thought that is probably forming in the back of your mind right now: *this sounds too simple to actually work.*

I understand that reaction completely. We're conditioned to believe that real solutions must be complicated, that healing requires intensive effort and specialized intervention, that anything this accessible and inexpensive can't be serious medicine.

But occasionally the most powerful interventions are the ones that address fundamental needs we've been ignoring. Your brain evolved outdoors. Your body evolved outdoors. For hundreds of thousands of years, humans lived entirely outside. Only in the most recent fraction of human history have we moved primarily indoors.

Going outside isn't a wellness trend or an alternative therapy. It's returning to a basic biological requirement—giving your brain and body access to the environment they were built for. The science is not ambiguous about this. The question is only whether you're willing to act on it.

You don't have to be convinced before you start. *You just have to be willing to try it.* Step outside tomorrow for twenty minutes. Not to exercise. Not to accomplish anything. Just to be outside and notice how you feel.

The chapters ahead will give you the science, the mechanisms, and the practical guidance to make outdoor time a real and lasting part of how you take care of yourself. But all of that starts with *one simple step out the door.*

Let's begin.

## References

American Society of Planning Officials. (1967, December). Vest pocket parks (Report No. 229). American Society of Planning Officials.

Berman, M. G., Jonides, J., & Kaplan, S. (2008). The cognitive benefits of interacting with nature. Psychological Science, 19(12), 1207–1212. https://doi.org/10.1111/j.1467-9280.2008.02225.x

Bratman, G. N., Hamilton, J. P., Hahn, K. S., Daily, G. C., & Gross, J. J. (2015). Nature experience reduces rumination and subgenual prefrontal cortex activation. Proceedings of the National Academy of Sciences, 112(28), 8567–8572. https://doi.org/10.1073/pnas.15104 59112

Fascitelli, Jack. (2019). *Robert Moses and the Real Estate City: A Reexamination of the Legacy of New York's Master Builder* [Documents]. Trinity Student Scholarship. Trinity College Digital Repository. https://jstor.org/stable/community.34031347

Hasan MK. Digital multitasking and hyperactivity: unveiling the hidden costs to brain health. Ann Med Surg (Lond). 2024 Sep 18;86(11):6371-6373. doi: 10.1097/MS9.0000000000002576 . PMID: 39525791; PMCID: PMC11543232.

Hunter, M. R., Gillespie, B. W., & Chen, S. Y. P. (2019). Urban nature experiences reduce stress in the context of daily life based on salivary biomarkers. Frontiers in Psychology, 10, 722. https://doi.or g/10.3389/fpsyg.2019.00722

Kaplan, R., & Kaplan, S. (1989). The experience of nature: A psychological perspective. Cambridge University Press.

Kaplan, S. (1995). The restorative benefits of nature: Toward an integrative framework. Journal of Environmental Psychology, 15(3), 169–182. https://doi.org/10.1016/0272-4944(95)90001-2

Park, B. J., Tsunetsugu, Y., Kasetani, T., Kagawa, T., & Miyazaki, Y. (2010). The physiological effects of Shinrin-yoku (taking in the forest atmosphere or forest bathing): Evidence from field experiments in 24 forests across Japan. Environmental Health and Preventive Medicine, 15(1), 18–26. https://doi.org/10.1007/s12199-009-0086-9

Schubert, D. (2019). Jane Jacobs, cities, urban planning, ethics and value systems. Cities, 91, 4-9. https://doi.org/10.1016/j.cities.2018.05.001

Ulrich, R. S., Simons, R. F., Losito, B. D., Fiorito, E., Miles, M. A., & Zelson, M. (1991). Stress recovery during exposure to natural and urban environments. Journal of Environmental Psychology, 11(3), 201–230. https://doi.org/10.1016/S0272-4944(05)80184-7

Walser, L. (2016, April 14). A tale of two planners: Jane Jacobs vs. Robert Moses. Saving Places. https://savingplaces.org/stories/a-tale-of-two-planners-jane-jacobs-and-robert-moses

White, M. P., Alcock, I., Grellier, J., Wheeler, B. W., Hartig, T., Warber, S. L., Bone, A., Depledge, M. H., & Fleming, L. E. (2019). Spending at least 120 minutes a week in nature is associated with good health and well-being. Scientific Reports, 9(1), 7730. https://doi.org/10.1038/s41598-019-44097-3

Wilson, E. O. (1984). Biophilia. Harvard University Press.

# Chapter 2: What Your Nose Knows: The Healing Power of Outdoor Scents

Here is something that rarely comes up in any conversation about mental health: ***how to breathe.***

Not deep-breathing exercises. Not the kind of slow inhales and the steady exhales you practice during a panic attack. Something different. Something simpler. Stepping outside, stopping for a moment, and just noticing what the air smells like.

*It sounds almost too small to matter.* But the research says otherwise. Your nose turns out to be *one of the most powerful therapeutic tools you own*—and you take it outside for free.

## The Scent That Calms You Down Before You Know It

You know that smell after it rains? That earthy, clean, slightly sweet smell that rises up from the ground after a good downpour? There's a word for it: ***petrichor.***

The word was only coined in the 1960s, but the experience is ancient. Scientists discovered that this scent comes from a combination of things happening at once—plant oils that have been building up in dry soil, compounds released by bacteria in the ground, and a molecule called geosmin that gets released when raindrops hit the earth. When rain strikes dry soil, it creates tiny aerosol particles that carry these scents up into the air, straight to your nose.

Breathing in forest VOCs (volatile organic compounds) can have helpful antioxidant and anti-inflammatory effects on our airways. Some, taken in through breathing, may also help brain functions by reducing mental tiredness, causing relaxation, and improving thinking and mood. The *types of trees can greatly affect the amount of certain VOCs in the forest air*, which also changes in daily cycles. Keep this in mind when you're thinking about where and what forest you may want to walk in.

And, the positive mental and physical effects of visiting a forest are not just from breathing in VOCs but come from a combined *stimulation of all five senses*, caused by all the special features of the natural environment, with sight likely playing a key role in the overall effect. This could be useful for personal well-being and public health.

Here's what the research tells us: smell doesn't just make you feel nostalgic. It actually *triggers relaxation in your brain*. Studies show that petrichor activates the limbic system—the *part of your brain responsible for emotions and memory*. People describe it as calming. Comforting. Like a signal that something good is coming.

Some scientists believe this response has evolutionary roots. Our ancestors depended on finding water. The smell of rain on dry ground may have been a cue—water is near, resources are coming, you can relax. Thousands of years later, your brain still gets that signal. You breathe in petrichor, and something in you quiets down before your conscious mind has even processed what happened.

Don't dismiss that. That's your nervous system doing exactly what it was designed to do.

## Pine Trees, Phytoncides, and Your Immune System

Pine trees—and many other conifers, along with oak, cedar, and cypress trees—release specific chemical compounds called *phytoncides.* The word literally means "plant secretions." Trees release these volatile organic compounds into the air around them, partly as a natural defense against insects and disease.

When you walk into a forest and breathe that sharp, resinous, alive smell, you're inhaling phytoncides. And your body responds to them in ways that researchers have also been documenting for decades. it's not your imagination at all because it's grounded in real specific science.

Dr. Qing Li at Nippon Medical School in Tokyo has some of the most compelling work in this area. In one study, he had participants take two-day trips into forests rich in Japanese cypress trees. Compared to people who spent the same time in an urban environment, the forest visitors showed significant *increases in natural killer cell activity*. Natural killer (NK) cells are *a crucial part of your immune system*—they identify and destroy cells that have become infected or cancerous. Those increases in NK cell activity *lasted for up to thirty days after the trip*.

Think about that. Two days in a pine forest produced immune benefits that **lasted a month**. The benefits are mind-boggling and it's almost like getting a natural vaccine.

*And it wasn't just being away from the city*. The researchers isolated the *specific phytoncides from the forest air*, put them in hotel rooms, and found that even sleeping in a room infused with these tree compounds produced measurable immune effects. *The forest's scent was doing the work.* Sounds like something they should be incorporating into those scented candles and oils they want us to buy for our homes, doesn't it? Or are they doing that?

For something as *accessible and free* as a walk in the woods, that's a remarkable return on investment. You don't need an appointment at a health care facility or a prescription because the forest is something waiting for you out there. All you have to do is pick up your feet and move into it. And it doesn't require that you pitch a tent and stay in the forest for a week or so. Look at how long those people were in the woods and how long the effect lasted. They got a benefit for a full month after just two days. Studies have shown that you don't need to remain for days in the forest to get the benefit; sometimes *only short trips into the woods or near the woods* will provide a strengthening of your immune system.

## What Forest Air Does to Your Stress Hormones

You already know from Chapter 1 that cortisol is your body's main stress hormone. High cortisol over time is associated with anxiety, depression, sleep problems, and a whole range of physical health issues. Lowering your cortisol levels is vital for your mental and physical health.

Here's where the scents of the outdoors come back in. A Japanese study looking specifically at *female college students who walked through a forest* found significant decreases in salivary cortisol levels compared to students who walked through an urban environment. By the end of the walk, their bodies had measurably reduced their stress response. And those researchers connected it directly to the scent profile of the forest—the soft woody smells, the damp earth, the cool air carrying plant compounds.

The mechanism seems to be through your parasympathetic nervous system—the brake pedal (the "pause" one) we talked about in Chapter 1. Forest scents appear to stimulate the parasympathetic response, nudging your body toward rest, recovery, and repair. Your heart rate slows. Your breathing deepens. Your muscles let go.

This is why people who have just come out of a forest often describe feeling as if they have slept without actually sleeping. Like something got reset. Like the noise in their head turned down a few notches.

It's real. The science backs it up. And it *starts with what you're breathing.* If walking presents a difficulty, all you have to do now is breathe and there's no walking involved, so *even someone with a mobility issue* can benefit here. Once again I'm reminded of all the patients who had tuberculosis and were taken to the hospital at Saranac Lake in upstate New York. They were placed outside, wrapped warmly in blankets and sat in the morning sun close to a forest. It truly was therapeutic; unfortunately, it didn't address the tuberculosis adequately, but it was a start.

## The Smell of Rain in Winter Is Different From the Smell of Summer

*Outdoor scents change with the seasons*, and those seasonal differences matter.

Researchers in Finland studied what happened when young adults were *exposed to a snow-covered forest landscape in winter.* Not just the sight of it—the whole experience, including the crisp, clean, cold air. Participants reported significantly better mood, greater psychological relaxation, and improved ability to focus their attention compared to people who had been in an urban environment. *Winter forests smell different from summer ones*—there's less biological activity, less decay, more of a clean mineral quality—but they're still restorative.

If you've ever stepped outside on a cold, clear morning and taken a deep breath—that almost sharp, startling freshness—you've experienced this. It's not just cold air. It's air that carries fewer pollutants, different moisture content, different compounds. And your body responds to it.

*Autumn has its own scent language*: the earthy smell of fallen leaves decomposing, the fungal notes from forest floors, the cooling of the air. Spring has the green smell of new growth, the sweetness of blossoms, the return of biological activity. *Each season has an olfactory signature*, and each one can have calming, restorative effects if you actually step outside and pay attention to it.

Psychiatric patients hospitalized in the Swiss Alps developed an intriguing change of symptoms in winter. The strong foehn winds that descended from the mountains during that season were theorized to have a negative impact on them. Exactly what was involved in the wind, in terms of their scent makeup, hasn't been studied extensively. As a psychology intern, I had a supervisor who wrote his dissertation on the fog that was regularly seen during specific times of the year. As he told me, the fog produced a noticeable increase in depression in individuals living there. Was it the fog or was it the fact that it became darker and they had less interaction with sunshine? This is an interesting question, which I don't believe he explored.

We've gotten so used to living in climate-controlled spaces that smell the same year-round—that slightly recycled, plastic-and-carpet indoor scent—that we've lost our relationship with the seasonal rhythms of the outdoor world. Getting that back doesn't require a wilderness expedition. *It just requires opening a door.*

## Your Nose Takes a Shortcut to Your Brain

Here's why scent is such a powerful therapeutic tool: *it has a direct line to the emotional center of your brain.*

Every other sense—sight, hearing, touch, taste—has to make a pit stop before it gets to the emotional parts of your brain. The signals travel through a relay station called the thalamus first, getting processed and sorted before they reach their destination.

*Smell is the exception*. Olfactory signals go straight from your nose to the *amygdala and hippocampus*—your brain's *centers for emotion and memory*—without that relay stop. This is why a smell or a scent can instantly produce a feeling or a memory before you've even consciously registered what you're smelling. It's why the smell of a grandparent's kitchen can transport you back to childhood in a fraction of a second. It's why the smell of a pine forest can produce a feeling of calm before your brain has a chance to explain why.

Your nose doesn't have to convince your brain that you're in a safe, calming environment. It just tells it directly. And your brain responds.

*For people dealing with anxiety*—where the challenge is often that the thinking brain gets overwhelmed by the emotional brain—this is significant. *Outdoor scents can soothe the emotional centers of your brain* through a pathway that bypasses the overthinking altogether. *You don't have to convince yourself to relax.* The forest air starts that process for you.

## What About Cities? What If You Can't Get to a Forest?

Fair point. So let's talk about urban scents and what we actually know about them.

*The first thing* to understand is that even *city parks* have some of these olfactory benefits. Trees in urban environments still release phytoncides. Soil in city parks still carries petrichor after rain. Community gardens smell like damp earth and growing things. Even a tree-lined street on a warm summer morning carries more olfactory information than anything you'll find indoors.

*The second thing* is that the research on smaller doses of outdoor exposure is encouraging. Studies show that even brief periods outside—twenty to thirty minutes—can produce measurable effects on stress hormones and mood. The effects are stronger in denser natural environments, but *something is always better than nothing.*

One practical approach: *use your nose deliberately.* Make use of its powerful ability to transmit sense directly to those important brain centers. When you're outside, stop moving for a moment and actually pay attention to what you smell. Most of us walk through outdoor environments looking at our phones or thinking about our to-do lists.

We're outside but not present. Try this approach instead: *step outside, close your eyes for thirty seconds, and just breathe.* Of course I'm not referring to you doing that if you are in an area where there is heavy traffic. This book aims to help, not hinder, your health. Notice what's in the air. The warmth, the coolness, the organic notes, the green smell after a mow or the rain smell after a storm. Let your nose do its job.

Okay, fair point. Being in a traffic-congested area is not going to work. Please be conscious of where you are and what you want to do to achieve the benefits you can get from breathing.

And for those days when getting outside really isn't possible? Researchers have looked at indoor approximations. Essential oils derived from cedarwood, pine, and cypress contain some of the same phytoncide compounds found in forest air. They're not the same as a real forest—the complexity of actual outdoor air can't be replicated in a bottle—but some studies have found modest benefits from diffusing these scents indoors during periods of stress. I recall that some researchers have even pointed to rooms in your home that may be paneled with natural woods that may provide this environmental stress reduction scent. If you're a fan of TV series, think of "Yellowstone," where the main house is completely unfinished wood. In fact, a number of architects are looking at designs for homes that use unfinished woods in certain areas to bring a more natural environmental element into the home or business. Since many people work from home these days, being in a room with natural wood might be quite helpful.

The goal, though, is *always the real thing*. Even a brief, intentional outdoor scent experience is more powerful than an indoor approximation.

## How to Use This in Your Daily Life

Here are the simplest ways to start using outdoor scents therapeutically:

**First,** make rain-smell moments intentional. When it rains—or right after it rains—go outside. Stand on your porch, walk around the block, just step out *for two minutes*. The petrichor compounds are most concentrated in those first minutes after rain hits dry soil. This is one of the easiest and most accessible scent therapy experiences available to almost anyone. Of course, anyone with any type of serious allergy problems should consult their health care professional before doing this.

**Second**, if you can get to any green space—a park, a trail, a community garden, even a block with mature trees—slow down and breathe. Don't just walk through it. Stop. Breathe through your nose. Give yourself *two or three minutes* to just be in the scent environment. You are, in a very literal way, letting nature do its work on you.

**Third**, pay attention to your seasonal scent experiences. The smell of leaves in autumn, the green freshness of spring, the crystalline cold of winter air—these are free therapeutic resources that most of us walk past without noticing. *Start noticing them.* As I write, spring is fully blooming. The large lawn in our complex has rapidly filled with violets and tiny wildflowers, all of which I'm sure are adding to the healthful scent in the environment.

**Fourth**, if you're using outdoor time as part of managing anxiety or stress, *try pairing your outdoor scent experience with slow breathing*. Breathe in slowly through your nose, hold for a moment, breathe out through your mouth. You're combining two calming mechanisms at once—the scent input and the breathing pattern. Both are activating your parasympathetic nervous system. Together, they're more powerful than either one alone.

Your nose knows things your brain hasn't caught up with yet. Start trusting it.

## References

Antonelli M, Donelli D, Barbieri G, Valussi M, Maggini V, Firenzuoli F. Forest Volatile Organic Compounds and Their Effects on Human Health: A State-of-the-Art Review. Int J Environ Res Public Health. 2020 Sep 7;17(18):6506. doi: 10.3390/ijerph17186506. PMID: 32906736; PMCID: PMC7559006.

Bear, I. J., & Thomas, R. G. (1964). Nature of argillaceous odor. Nature, 201(4923), 993–995. https://www.nature.com/articles/201993a0

Bielinis, E., et al. (2021). The effects of viewing a winter forest landscape with the ground and trees covered in snow on the psychological relaxation of young Finnish adults: A pilot study. PLOS ONE. https://doi.org/10.1371/journal.pone.0258856

Li, Q. (2010). Effect of forest bathing trips on human immune function. Environmental Health and Preventive Medicine, 15(1), 9–17. https://doi.org/10.1007/s12199-008-0068-3

Matsunaga, K., et al. (2011). Aromatic effects of a Japanese forest on mood and stress in female university students. International Journal of Environmental Research and Public Health, 8(9), 3532–3542. https://www.mdpi.com/1660-4601/8/9/3532

Mikutta CA, Pervilhac C, Znoj H, Federspiel A, Müller TJ. The Impact of Foehn Wind on Mental Distress among Patients in a Swiss Psychiatric Hospital. Int J Environ Res Public Health. 2022 Aug 30;19(17):10831. doi: 10.3390/ijerph191710831. PMID: 36078547; PMCID: PMC9518389.

Morita, E., Fukuda, S., Nagano, J., Hamajima, N., Yamamoto, H., Iwai, Y., Nakashima, T., Ohira, H., & Shirakawa, T. (2007). Psychological effects of forest environments on healthy adults: Shinrin-yoku (forest-air bathing, or walking) as a possible method of stress reduction. Public Health, 121(1), 54–63. https://doi.org/10.1016/j.puhe.2006.05.024

Neff, E.P. Stop and smell the geosmin. Lab Anim 47, 270 (2018). https://doi.org/10.1038/s41684-018-0161-1

Shampo MA, Kyle RA, Steensma DP. Edward L. Trudeau--founder of a sanatorium for treatment of tuberculosis. Mayo Clin Proc. 2010 Jul;85(7):e48. doi: 10.4065/mcp.2010.0379. PMID: 20592164; PMCID: PMC2894729.

Tsunetsugu, Y., Park, B. J., & Miyazaki, Y. (2010). Trends in research related to 'Shinrin-yoku' (taking in the forest atmosphere or forest bathing) in Japan. Environmental Health and Preventive Medicine, 15(1), 27–37. https://doi.org/10.1007/s12199-009-0091-z

Uebi, T., et al. (2021). Geosmin triggers a pleasant neural response in humans. Frontiers in Neuroscience, 15. https://www.frontiersin.org/articles/10.3389/fnins.2021.674394/full

# Chapter 3: Blue Mind: Why Water Changes Everything

There is something that happens to people when they get near water. Perhaps that's why so many people plan their vacations near the water or on the water.

It doesn't matter much what kind of water. The ocean. A lake. A river. A pond in a city park. Even a fountain in a courtyard. People slow down. Their voices soften. They stop checking their phones. They just... look.

If you've felt this yourself, you probably assumed it was just personal preference—that you happen to like water. But it isn't personal preference. It's biology. And the research on what water does to the human brain and body is *some of the most compelling in the entire field of nature and mental health.*

## What Scientists Call Blue Mind

Marine biologist Wallace J. Nichols coined the term "*blue mind*" to describe the mildly meditative state that humans enter when they're near, in, on, or even under water. It's not a poetic description. It's a functional one. Nichols gathered neuroscientists, psychologists, and researchers from multiple fields to study this phenomenon, and what they found was consistent: *proximity to water produces measurable changes in brain activity, stress hormones, and emotional state.* That's pretty astounding, considering it's just the water being there.

The opposite of blue mind, Nichols says, is "*red mind*"—the state most of us live in most of the time. *Overstimulated. Overconnected. Anxious. Distracted.* Slightly overwhelmed by the sheer volume of information, decisions, and demands flooding our brains every day. Possibly think of it as being on fire most of the time from everything that is being demanded of you and all of the stress it entails.

Water interrupts that pattern. It gives your brain something to focus on that requires almost no effort—the movement, the sound, the light on the surface. This is the same "*soft fascination*" we talked about in Chapter 1, the kind that restores your attention system without draining it. Water is particularly effective at producing this state because it *engages multiple senses at once*: the sound of moving water, the visual complexity of waves or ripples, the smell of a lake or ocean, the cool of the air near the surface. One of my favorite childhood memories was when we were driving somewhere near the coast and you could smell the ocean air. It was exciting because I was thinking about how wonderful the ocean and the beach. Nice memory .

Your brain gets absorbed without getting taxed. And that's when the healing happens.

## The Sound of Water and Your Nervous System

You don't even have to see water to get some of its benefits. *The sound alone does something to your brain.*

Research has found that the sound of flowing water—rivers, streams, rain, ocean waves—activates the parasympathetic nervous system, the same "*rest and digest*" system we talked about in Chapter 1. It slows your heart rate. It deepens your breathing. It lowers your cortisol levels. all this from just hearing the sounds of water?

Scientists believe this response is *deeply evolutionary*. Moving water in the natural world is almost always a signal of something good: a clean water source, a livable environment, and safety. Our brains evolved to respond to that signal with relief. When you hear water, some ancient part of your brain registers: "*We're okay. We're near resources. We can rest.*"

That's why *recordings of ocean waves and rain are among the most popular sleep and relaxation aids* ever created. They're not just pleasant—they're activating a biological response that's been wired into you for hundreds of thousands of years. Do a simple internet search and you'll find audio of soothing water sounds that you can put on your computer and use whenever you need a stress break. Many are free and some are subscription services. ***The Internet Archive*** has a collection of 78 water sounds that you can download and then decide which ones are best for you ***and they're free.***

## Living Near Water and Mental Health

One of the most striking findings in this area comes from *large-scale population studies* looking at who lives near water and how healthy they are. One thing to remember whenever you're looking at research is *the size of the population that was examined.* Small populations may show important factors, but they can't be used to draw conclusions about a population that may be in the tens of thousands or even millions.

A major study published in Health and Place analyzed health data from *over 48 million people in England* and found that those who lived near the coast reported significantly better mental health than those who lived farther inland—even after *controlling for income, employment, and other factors*. The researchers found a *clear "blue space" effect*, separate from the green space effect of parks and forests. We're getting into *several different spaces,* each one with a color associated with it: ***blue, red, and green***.

A separate study published in Environmental Research found that people who lived within a kilometer of the coast were *22 percent less likely to report symptoms of depression or anxiety* than people who lived farther away. What would account for this if they were living near the coast but not on the coast? It might be what's in the air from the water on the coast that is drifting to them. Not just one factor here regarding being near the water because there are multiple other factors that are associated with near-water environments.

*These aren't small effects*. And they don't require you to live on the coast or own a boat. Other research has shown similar, though somewhat smaller, effects for people who live near rivers, lakes, and other inland bodies of water. *Any consistent proximity to water appears to provide mental health benefits.*

## What Happens When You Actually Get In

Being near water helps. *Being in water does something more.*

Cold water immersion—sometimes called cold water swimming or wild swimming—has attracted serious scientific attention in recent years. The research is consistent enough that it's worth looking at carefully.

A systematic review published in PLOS ONE in 2025 analyzed the available research on cold water immersion and found *significant psychological benefits: reduced depression and anxiety symptoms, improved mood, and better overall sense of wellbeing*. The effects weren't minor. Some participants in the studies reported that cold water swimming had more impact on their mental health than medication or therapy—though researchers are careful to note that it *works best as a complement to other treatment, not a replacement.* we need to remember that it's not just being in the water. Usually, when we're in the water, we are engaging in some type of exercise, such as swimming or even floating. And wait until you learn what muscles can do. We're going to deal with that in Chapter 5, where you will see muscles are more than you ever thought.

Do you know what famous Hollywood icon went swimming every day in the cold waters off Long Island Sound? The actress Katharine Hepburn said she couldn't go a day without swimming in the bay near her home. Yes, she swam regardless of the season. And she wasn't alone in believing that cold water had benefits. A very famous and exclusive boys' school in Great Britain, where the future kings were educated, always had the students take cold showers in the morning. I suppose they believed that this would make the students more alert. Who wouldn't be alert after a cold shower?

What's happening physiologically is that cold water immersion triggers a strong activation of your sympathetic nervous system—the "fight or flight" response—followed by a shift into parasympathetic recovery. Your body releases norepinephrine and other *neurochemicals associated with alertness, mood elevation, and reduced pain.* Over time, regular cold water exposure appears to train your stress response to be more flexible—*quicker to activate and quicker to recover.* As for me, I will forego the cold showers.

Again, a narrative review in the International Journal of Environmental Research and Public Health found that *cold water swimming* was associated with improvements in mood, energy, confidence, and pain tolerance. Participants described feeling more alive, more present, and more resilient after regular cold water exposure. I'm not espousing that you begin swimming in cold water, only reporting what the research indicates.

## You Don't Have to Go Polar

Before you close this book: *you do not need to plunge into a frozen lake to benefit from water.*

The research on cold water immersion is compelling, but the benefits of water exposure *exist on a spectrum*. *A cool shower* has documented effects on *mood and alertness*. **Sitting** by a stream for twenty minutes has measurable *effects on cortisol*. **Walking** along a beach—even without going in the water—produces significant reductions in stress.

The principle is simply that water—in almost any form you can access—gives your nervous system something it responds to deeply. It's one of the most effective and accessible natural interventions for stress, anxiety, and low mood that the research has identified. Yes, it's primitive but we have primitive areas within our brain. In fact, one *portion of the brain is referred to as the reptilian brain*.

If you live near water of any kind—a river, a lake, a pond, a beach, even a fountain in a park—you have a resource most people don't think to use. *Start using it.*

## Water, Weather, and the Winter Season

One thing worth knowing: *water in winter is not off-limits.*

Winter swimming has a long tradition in Scandinavian and Eastern European cultures, and the research on it is fascinating. A study published in Biochemia Medica found that regular winter swimmers showed *positive changes in blood chemistry* and reported significantly better mood and energy levels than non-swimmers. Participants reported feeling invigorated, less fatigued, and more emotionally stable.

You don't need to adopt a year-round cold-water practice to get something from water in winter. Standing by a river on a cold morning, listening to the sound of moving water, breathing the cool clean air near the surface—these experiences are *available to almost anyone, in almost any season*, at almost no cost.

The water is there. It has been there for your entire species' history. Your brain knows exactly what to do when you get near it.

## How to Bring Water Into Your Mental Health Practice

Here are practical ways to start using water as a therapeutic resource:

**First**, find your nearest water. This might be an ocean beach, a river trail, a lakeside park, or just a fountain in a public square. Make a point of knowing where it is. Then *make a point of going.*

**Second**, when you get there, *slow down*. Don't just walk past the water. *Stop. Sit* near it if you can. Let your eyes track the movement on the surface. *Listen. Breathe*. Give it at least *ten minutes* before you start checking your phone. The benefits build over time.

**Third**, if you're open to it, consider getting in. You don't have to start with cold. Even swimming in a warm lake or pool outdoors provides the combination of water immersion, natural environment, and physical movement that the research identifies as particularly powerful for mood. If you want to explore cold water, start small—a slightly cooler shower, a brief wade in cool water—and work up gradually. Everyone is different, and everyone has different tolerances and needs. *We're not asking you to exceed any of these*, or to feel that you have been a failure if you can't progress beyond a certain point. That's you, and you should be satisfied with it. The major thing here is to *give it a try*. It's not for you; that's fine.

**Fourth**, *use water sound intentionally* on days when you can't get outside. Recordings of rain, rivers, and ocean waves have documented calming effects. They're not the same as the real thing, but on a difficult day, they're a resource. Think of it this way: how we used to think of seasonal vegetables when we didn't have access to foods grown all over the world and depended on the seasons for our food. When that wasn't possible, we went to canned or frozen foods. We'd still like the real thing but when that's not possible, you can go to an alternative.

Water has been central to human life and human health for as long as humans have existed. *Going back to it isn't a trend. It's a return, like being in a place that once was very familiar to us.*

## References

Cain, D., et al. (2025). Cold-water immersion: Systematic review of physiological and psychological effects. PLOS ONE. https://journals.plos.org/plosone/article?id=10.1371/journal.pone.0292321

Cracknell, D., White, M. P., Pahl, S., Nichols, W. J., & Depledge, M. H. (2016). Marine nature experience and its significance to well-being: A qualitative study. International Journal of Wellbeing, 6(1). https://doi.org/10.5502/ijw.v6i1.497

Knechtle, B., et al. (2020). Cold water swimming—benefits and risks: A narrative review. International Journal of Environmental Research and Public Health, 17(23), 8984. https://www.mdpi.com/1660-4601/17/23/8984

Naumann RK, Ondracek JM, Reiter S, Shein-Idelson M, Tosches MA, Yamawaki TM, Laurent G. The reptilian brain. Curr Biol. 2015 Apr 20;25(8):R317-21. doi: 10.1016/j.cub.2015.02.049. PMID: 25898097; PMCID: PMC4406946.

Nichols, W. J. (2014). Blue mind: The surprising science that shows how being near, in, on, or under water can make you happier, healthier, more connected, and better at what you do. Little, Brown and Company.

Sińczuk, M., et al. (2011). Effects of winter swimming on hematological parameters. Biochemia Medica. https://doi.org/10.11613/BM.2011.035

Wheeler, B. W., White, M., Stahl-Timmins, W., & Depledge, M. H. (2012). Does living by the coast improve health and well-being? Health and Place, 18(5), 1198–1201. https://doi.org/10.1016/j.healthplace.2012.06.015

White, M. P., Alcock, I., Wheeler, B. W., & Depledge, M. H. (2013). Would you be happier living in a greener urban area? A fixed-effects analysis of panel data. Psychological Science, 24(6), 920–928. https://doi.org/10.1177/0956797612464659

# Chapter 4: Let There Be Light: What Sunlight Actually Does to Your Brain

Here is a question worth sitting with: *When was the last time you spent a full hour in natural outdoor light?* And please, when I say natural outdoor light, I'm talking about sunshine, of course, but you don't go out there without some sunscreen protection.

Not through a window. Not in a sunroom. **Outside**, with actual sunlight falling on your skin and your eyes open to the real sky.

If you have to think hard to remember, you're not alone. Most of us spend our days under artificial light—the flat, steady glow of LED bulbs and fluorescent tubes—and we have stopped noticing that it's not the same thing as sunlight. Not even close. And *our brains are paying a price for that* substitution that most of us *have never been told about.*

Yes, there's a price but there's also something you need to do if you are going to be sitting in direct sunlight: As I said, wear sunscreen to protect yourself. We know that while sunlight is beneficial, too much of it can also cause skin cancer, and we don't want that to happen. Even those with dark skin are vulnerable to skin cancer, despite the myth that they are protected from it. It's a deadly disease. If you have *certain illnesses like lupus,* being in direct sunlight can produce adverse physical effects, even stroke.

This chapter is about light. What it does to your brain, why it matters for your mood and your sleep and your ability to function, and why getting outside to experience real daylight—*especially in the morning*—may be one of the most powerful free tools you have for mental health.

## Your Brain Runs on a Clock You Cannot Override

Inside your brain, in a region called the hypothalamus, there is a tiny cluster of cells roughly *the size of a grain of rice*. It is called the suprachiasmatic nucleus. Most people have never heard of it. But it runs your life more than almost anything else in your body. Interestingly, it's also the small organic mechanism that helps birds find their way when they are in flight or migrating, although we have to wonder how albatrosses use it since they are *able to fly while asleep.*

This cluster of cells is *your biological clock.* It governs what scientists call your circadian rhythm—the roughly 24-hour cycle that controls when you feel awake and alert, when you feel sleepy, when your body releases stress hormones, when your temperature rises and falls, and dozens of other functions. *Every cell in your body follows the rhythm set by this tiny clock.* I've had at least one sleep researcher, a very famous one at that, tell me we don't run on a 24-hour cycle but a 25-hour cycle. I haven't seen anything in the literature about that 25-hour cycle. What they have indicated is that the cycle is 12 minutes longer than 24 hours but not 25.

And that clock is calibrated—reset every single day—by light. Specifically, by *natural outdoor light entering your eyes in the morning.* The best time to reset it? In early morning light.

This is not optional. It is not a preference. It is a biological requirement. Your circadian clock needs that light signal to stay accurate, the way a watch needs to be wound or to recharge when it's a solar watch by placing it in the sun. When it doesn't get that input—when you spend your mornings indoors under artificial light, or you never step outside in the early hours—***the clock drifts***. And when the clock drifts, almost everything it controls starts to go wrong.

Researchers Charles Czeisler and John Gooley at Harvard Medical School have spent decades documenting this relationship between light and the biological clock. Their work shows that *morning light exposure sets the timing* for daily cycles of alertness and emotional well-being—and that disrupting this natural signal through *shift work, irregular schedules, or simply staying indoors* can increase the risk of mood swings and depression. The clock is not a metaphor. It is a real physical mechanism. And it needs light to function properly.

## Why Indoor Light Is Not Enough

You may be thinking, *I have plenty of light in my home. My office is well-lit. My screens are bright. Doesn't that count?*

**It doesn't.** And the reason is *intensity.*

Light is measured in units called lux. On a bright sunny day outdoors, light intensity reaches around 100,000 lux. On a cloudy overcast day, it is still somewhere between 10,000 and 30,000 lux. *A well-lit office? Typically 300 to 500 lux.* A brightly lit living room might reach 1,000 on a good day. Consider how significant the difference is between a sunny day (**100,000 lux**) and your indoor office (**300 to 500 lux**). There is no question in anybody's mind that there must be a similarly significant difference in how those *two different types of light affect you.*

Your brain's light-sensing system—particularly the *specialized cells in your eyes* that calibrate your circadian clock—requires exposure to high-lux light to do its job. The difference between outdoor light and indoor light is not subtle. It is enormous. Your brain knows the difference even when your conscious mind doesn't register it. Did you know that our eyes are considered the *stalks of the brain* so they can transmit information directly to the brain?

This is why people who work entirely indoors often describe feeling foggy, flat, or off in ways they can't quite explain. Their biological clocks are not getting the signal they need. The lights are on, but not the right kind of on. Numerous studies have also examined shift workers and the incidence of depression, anxiety, and even physical illness that may be associated with their lack of exposure to natural daylight. It's not just the circadian rhythm that is upset; it's also physical factors that are affected by this disruption, and some have suggested *it may even be associated with higher rates of diabetes and cancer.* If getting out in the sun is important, this research indicates there is a dire need for it in order to maintain optimal health.

## Sunlight, Serotonin, and Why You Feel Better Outside

Serotonin is one of the brain's most important chemical messengers. It plays a central role in mood, emotional stability, and the quiet, steady feeling of well-being that makes a good day feel enjoyable. Low serotonin activity is linked to depression, anxiety, irritability, and poor impulse control. Many of the most widely prescribed antidepressants—the SSRIs—work specifically by keeping serotonin available in the brain for longer. You may be interested to know that the brain is highly efficient at *recycling these chemical messengers* once they are used, bringing them back, repackaging them, and reusing them. It's called *reuptake (the pineal gland is involved).*

Here is what most people don't know: *sunlight directly stimulates serotonin production*. When bright light enters your eyes, it triggers a pathway that increases the release of serotonin in your brain. Researchers have found that serotonin levels in the brain track closely with the amount of sunlight on any given day—higher on bright days, lower on dim ones.

A landmark study published in The Lancet measured serotonin production directly and found that serotonin turnover in the brain was significantly higher on days with more bright sunlight. The effect was *independent of temperature and season*. It was the light itself doing the work, not the warmth, not the calendar. When sunlight hits your eyes, your brain produces more of the chemical that underlies stable mood. It's that direct.

This is part of why people consistently report feeling better when they go outside—even when they didn't expect to, even when they were reluctant to go. It isn't just a change of scenery. *It's a biochemical shift*. Your brain is receiving the signal it was designed to receive, producing the neurochemical it was designed to produce, which is vital for stabilizing our mood.

## Vitamin D: The Sunlight Nutrient Most of Us Are Missing

There is a second pathway through which sunlight affects your health, and *it runs through your skin* rather than your eyes.

When ultraviolet light from the sun hits your skin, *your body produces vitamin D*. You may have heard of vitamin D mainly in the context of bone health—and it matters enormously for your bones. But the research has expanded considerably since those early findings. Vitamin D receptors exist in virtually every tissue in the body, including the brain. Low vitamin D levels have been consistently linked to higher rates of depression, anxiety, and cognitive decline.

Michael Holick at Boston University Medical Center has spent decades studying vitamin D and its role in human health. His work and the research that has followed show that vitamin D deficiency is far more common than most people realize—particularly in northern climates, in people who work indoors, and in darker-skinned individuals whose skin requires more sun exposure to produce the same amount of vitamin D. Estimates suggest that somewhere between 40 and 50 percent of American adults are vitamin D deficient or insufficient. The mental health consequences of that deficiency are real and measurable.

Getting *outside for even twenty to thirty minutes during midday hours*—when the sun's angle is high enough for your skin to produce vitamin D—addresses two things at once: the eye-based light signal that calibrates your biological clock, and the skin-based production of a nutrient your brain needs to function well. So, it's a two-for-one win-win for you.

## Seasonal Affective Disorder: What It Tells Us About Everyone

You have probably heard of seasonal affective disorder, or SAD. It is the form of depression that arrives with the shorter, darker days of autumn and winter and typically lifts in spring. Most people don't know that there is a second form of seasonal affective disorder that people *experience during the summer months,* not in the winter as we had previously thought.

Roughly 10 million Americans experience SAD every year, and many more experience a milder version—sometimes called the winter blues—that doesn't rise to the level of clinical depression but still makes life noticeably harder. Energy drops. Motivation fades. Sleep becomes heavy. Getting out of bed feels like work.

SAD is essentially what happens when the circadian clock *doesn't get sufficient light to function properly for weeks or months at a time.* The days shorten, the light grows weaker, and the biological clock loses its calibration. Serotonin production drops. Melatonin—the hormone that signals darkness and induces sleep—lingers longer into the morning hours. The body gets confused about what time it is, and mood and energy suffer accordingly.

Researchers Roecklein and Rohan, who have reviewed the SAD literature extensively, describe it as one of the clearest demonstrations that human beings are biological creatures with biological needs—and that *light is one of those fundamental needs, not an extra.* When we don't get enough of it, predictable things go wrong.

But here is why SAD matters even if you don't personally experience it in its full form: it is the extreme end of a spectrum that affects nearly everyone. Most people feel somewhat flatter, heavier, and less motivated in winter than in summer. Their energy and mood respond to light in ways they have probably never thought of as biological. The lesson of SAD research is not just that some people have a serious condition. It is that all of us are light-dependent creatures, and all of us *function better with more outdoor light exposure* than we are currently getting.

## Morning Is the Critical Window

Not all sunlight exposure is equally valuable. The timing matters—and the research is consistent about when that window opens.

Morning light, in the *first one to two hours after waking*, has a disproportionate effect on the biological clock compared to light received later in the day. The reasons have to do with the angle of light in the early hours, the spectrum it carries, and the way the circadian system is designed to receive its daily calibration signal at the start of the day rather than midday or evening.

When you get outdoor light exposure in the morning, you are doing several things at once. You are *clearing the melatonin* that makes you feel groggy and slow. You are *triggering the serotonin pathways* that support positive, stable mood. And you are *setting the timing of your biological clock* so that it will release melatonin again at the right time that night, making it easier to fall asleep. A good morning of outdoor light creates a better night of sleep, which creates a better morning the next day. It is a *self-reinforcing cycle*—but you have to be the one to start it.

I can tell you, from personal experience, that simply walking to my car outside for five minutes, after removing my baseball cap for protection, it gave me a decided lift in my mood and outlook for the day. I know the idea sounds incredibly simplistic, but I experienced it. Despite the pooh-poohing of personal experience over experiments, it's real. I have experienced it, and I know others can experience it, too. It didn't take long and the change happened in not minutes but seconds. Give it a try. Isn't your health and your mood worth a few minutes? Just five minutes or less. If you find the idea of spending hours outdoors too much for you, think about my experience. Even a few minutes of outdoor sunshine can contribute greatly to you.

A large cohort study that *tracked over 300,000 people* in the UK for approximately twelve years found that spending one to two hours per day in outdoor sunlight was associated with the lowest risk of depression—regardless of the genetic factors that might otherwise predispose someone to mental health challenges. Below that daily threshold, depression risk climbed. The numbers were not ambiguous. More outdoor daylight, especially in the morning, correlated directly with better mental health outcomes across a very large population over a very long time.

If we think back not that many years in medical history, we can remember that patients with tuberculosis, as well as individuals in rehab facilities or nursing homes, were, whenever possible, placed outside in the sunshine in the morning, either on terraces or on lawns.

## What About Skin Safety?

This is a fair question, and it deserves a straight answer.

The concern about sun exposure and skin cancer is real. Excessive UV exposure—particularly the kind that causes sunburn—does increase the risk of skin cancer. That is not in dispute. Severe sunburns in childhood can later in life return to be pre-cancerous growths (AK) or even skin cancer known as melanoma.

But the research on the benefits of outdoor light is *not asking you to sunbathe for hours or to ignore sun protection*. It is asking you to get outside for *twenty to thirty minutes,* particularly in the morning hours when the UV index is lower. Anyone of a certain age will remember a rock song that talked about going out in the midday sun and who was the only one who did it. Morning light provides the eye-based signals that calibrate your biological clock and stimulate serotonin with minimal UV risk, because the sun is lower in the sky and UV intensity is lower at that angle. Skin-based vitamin D production requires somewhat more exposure at higher sun angles, but the recommended amounts are still modest—*fifteen to twenty minutes* of midday exposure on arms and legs, *a few times a week*, is enough for most people.

The practical guidance is simple: get outside in the morning, without sunglasses if you can safely do so for a short period, because your eyes need direct light input for the circadian signal. Use sun protection during extended midday exposure. The goal is not to maximize sun time. It is to get the minimum effective dose that your biological systems need—which most of us are currently getting far less of than required.

## Light Therapy: When You Cannot Get Enough Natural Light

For people who live in northern latitudes, work night shifts, or genuinely cannot get outside consistently during daylight hours, light therapy offers a well-researched alternative.

A light therapy box produces light in the range of 10,000 lux—roughly equivalent to outdoor light on a bright overcast day—and is *used for twenty to thirty minutes in the morning.* Dozens of well-designed studies have found that morning light therapy reduces symptoms of SAD, improves mood, helps recalibrate disrupted sleep schedules, and increases daytime alertness. It is one of the most evidence-based tools in the mental health toolkit, and it is available without a prescription for around fifty dollars. Remember another fact: not everyone can tolerate being in front of one of these boxes. Some people can develop a sunburn. *You should consult with a dermatologist* before you begin using any of these boxes and ask for recommendations *or whether you are a candidate to use them at all.*

Allow me to once again repeat a caution. Light therapy is *not a substitute for actual outdoor time*—the full experience of being outside involves more than just lux levels. But for the days when getting outside is genuinely not possible, a light therapy box used in the morning provides a meaningful version of the signal your brain is looking for.

## How to Make Light Work for You Every Day

The practical changes here are among the simplest in this book, because they don't require equipment or a particular destination. They require only that you step outside at the right time.

**First,** make outdoor morning light non-negotiable. Not for exercise. Not to accomplish anything. Just for light. Ten to fifteen minutes outside within the first hour of waking—walking, sitting, standing on a porch—gives your biological clock the signal it needs. If it is cloudy, go anyway. *Overcast outdoor light may provide more lux than indoor light.* The signal gets through even through clouds.

**Second**, avoid sunglasses during your morning light time if you can safely do so. The circadian signal depends on light entering your eyes. Sunglasses reduce that input significantly. Morning sun angles are generally low enough that short unprotected exposure carries minimal risk—but use your own judgment based on conditions.

**Third,** if your lunch break is your only reliable outdoor time, protect it. Twenty minutes outside at midday provides a serotonin boost, a brief reset of the attention system, and vitamin D-producing UV light. It is one of the most accessible mental health practices available to almost anyone with a door to step through.

**Fourth**, notice what happens when you are consistent across the seasons. Winter mornings are darker and the light is weaker, but outdoor time remains more effective than staying inside. Most people who make morning outdoor time a consistent habit in the colder months—rather than giving it up when the weather turns—notice a real difference in their energy and mood by the second week.

The light has always been out there. *You just have to step into it.*

## References

Cassone VM, Paulose JK, Whitfield-Rucker MG, Peters JL. Time's arrow flies like a bird: two paradoxes for avian circadian biology. Gen Comp Endocrinol. 2009 Sep 1;163(1-2):109-16. doi: 10.1016/j.ygcen.2009.01.003. Epub 2009 Jan 23. PMID: 19523398; PMCID: PMC2710421.

Czeisler, C. A., & Gooley, J. J. (2007). Sleep and circadian rhythms in humans. Cold Spring Harbor Symposia on Quantitative Biology, 72, 579–597. https://doi.org/10.1101/sqb.2007.72.064

Dennis LK, Vanbeek MJ, Beane Freeman LE, Smith BJ, Dawson DV, Coughlin JA. Sunburns and risk of cutaneous melanoma: does age matter? A comprehensive meta-analysis. Ann Epidemiol. 2008 Aug;18(8):614-27. doi: 10.1016/j.annepidem.2008.04.006. PMID: 18652979; PMCID: PMC2873840.

Holick, M. F. (2004). Vitamin D: Importance in the prevention of cancers, type 1 diabetes, heart disease, and osteoporosis. American Journal of Clinical Nutrition, 79(3), 362–371. https://academic.oup.com/ajcn/article/79/3/362/4690087

Holick, M. F. (2007). Vitamin D deficiency. New England Journal of Medicine, 357(3), 266–281. https://doi.org/10.1056/NEJMra070553

Kim A, Chong BF. Photosensitivity in cutaneous lupus erythematosus. Photodermatol Photoimmunol Photomed. 2013 Feb;29(1):4-11. doi: 10.1111/phpp.12018. PMID: 23281691; PMCID: PMC3539182.

Klein, D. C. (2016). The pineal gland and melatonin. In J. L. Jameson & L. J. De Groot (Eds.), Endocrinology: Adult and pediatric (7th ed., pp. 312–322). W.B. Saunders. https://doi.org/10.1016/B978-0-323-18907-1.00019-6

Lambert, G. W., Reid, C., Kaye, D. M., Jennings, G. L., & Esler, M. D. (2002). Effect of sunlight and season on serotonin turnover in the brain. The Lancet, 360(9348), 1840–1842. https://doi.org/10.1016/S0140-6736(02)11737-5

Meesters Y, Gordijn MC. Seasonal affective disorder, winter type: current insights and treatment options. Psychol Res Behav Manag. 2016 Nov 30;9:317-327. doi: 10.2147/PRBM.S114906. PMID: 27942239; PMCID: PMC5138072

Melrose S. Seasonal Affective Disorder: An Overview of Assessment and Treatment Approaches. Depress Res Treat.

2015;2015:178564. doi: 10.1155/2015/178564. Epub 2015 Nov 25. PMID: 26688752; PMCID: PMC4673349.

Nguyen CTO, Acosta ML, Di Angelantonio S, Salt TE. Editorial: Seeing Beyond the Eye: The Brain Connection. Front Neurosci. 2021 Jun 29;15:719717. doi: 10.3389/fnins.2021.719717. PMID: 34267626; PMCID: PMC8276094.

Pail, G., Huf, W., Pjrek, E., Winkler, D., Willeit, M., Praschak-Rieder, N., & Kasper, S. (2011). Bright-light therapy in the treatment of mood disorders. Neuropsychobiology, 64(3), 152–162. https://doi.org/10.1159/000328950

Purves D, Augustine GJ, Fitzpatrick D, et al., editors. Neuroscience. 2nd edition. Sunderland (MA): Sinauer Associates; 2001. Neurotransmitter Release and Removal. Available from: https://www.ncbi.nlm.nih.gov/books/NBK11106/

Rattenborg, N., Voirin, B., Cruz, S. et al. Evidence that birds sleep in mid-flight. Nat Commun 7, 12468 (2016). https://doi.org/10.1038/ncomms12468

Roecklein, K. A., & Rohan, K. J. (2005). Seasonal affective disorder: An overview and update. Psychiatry, 2(1), 20–26. https://pubmed.ncbi.nlm.nih.gov/23878527/

Shaffer, J. A., Bhatt, D. L., & Bhatt, N. (2022). Outdoor time and mental health: Large-scale analysis of daylight exposure and depression risk. JAMA Psychiatry, 79(4), 330–339. https://jamanetwork.com/journals/jamapsychiatry/fullarticle/2789493

Shidhore N, Mangot A. Sunshine and Sadness: A Case Report on Summer Season Depression. Cureus. 2024 Dec 5;16(12):e75190. doi: 10.7759/cureus.75190. PMID: 39759719; PMCID: PMC11700541.

Tähkämö, L., Partonen, T., & Pesonen, A. K. (2019). Systematic review of light exposure impact on human circadian rhythm.

Chronobiology International, 36(2), 151–170. https://doi.org/10.1080/07420528.2018.1527773

UCLA Health. (2022). Being in natural light improves mood, increases happiness. UCLA Health. https://www.uclahealth.org/news/being-in-natural-light-improves-mood-increases-happiness

Wijaya, L. N., & Makiyah, S. N. N. (2020). Effects Of Sunlight Exposure For Treatment of Tuberculosis: Literature Review. Journal Of Nursing Practice, 3(2), 123–131. https://doi.org/10.30994/jnp.v3i2.78

Xu M, Yin X, Gong Y. Lifestyle Factors in the Association of Shift Work and Depression and Anxiety. JAMA Netw Open. 2023;6(8):e2328798. doi:10.1001/jamanetworkopen.2023.28798

# Chapter 5: Move Your Body, Heal Your Mind: The Science of Green Exercise

## The Workout You're Not Getting at the Gym

Let me ask you something. When you think about exercise for mental health, *what comes to mind?* Probably a gym. Maybe a treadmill. Or the image of someone running on a track or lifting weights in a brightly lit room with mirrors on every wall. *That's what we've been sold*. Get your heart rate up, burn some calories, get your dopamine hit, and go home. What it really all boils down to is marketing. You've been sold a bill of goods that isn't the best one for you. Undoubtedly, exercise is good wherever you do it, but there's a better place than the gym to do it. There is one thing more that I need to contribute to this book about muscles and it is of great importance.

Most of us think of muscles as biological rubber bands that hold our joints together and help us move in the ways we intend. Muscles *have another function* that was discovered only within the past two decades: **they are endocrine glands, too.** As such, they are more than elastic bands because they are the signal providers for so many functions in the body. We have yet to discover all of them. What are some of them?

Muscles produce and secrete signaling molecules called myokines, enabling communication between muscle and various organs, including the brain, adipose tissue (fat), bone, liver, gut, pancreas, blood vessels, and skin. In addition, myokines regulate metabolism, inflammation, and energy balance. Others include myostatin (regulates muscle growth). That's not all they do because muscles also have additional functions and benefits to us.

During exercise, *muscles release IL-6 into the bloodstream*, which then acts *on the liver to regulate glucose production*, on adipose tissue to *stimulate fat breakdown*, and *on the immune system* to reduce inflammation. It is a multifunctional cytokine that acts as both a pro-inflammatory signal and an anti-inflammatory myokine.

This may sound a bit confusing or too deep, I know. What you need to take away from this discussion is that exercise and working our muscles *has an effect on everything involved in good health, including maintaining good cognition* because it **affects the brain**. A bit of simple exercise and look what your muscles are doing for you. It's incredible.

No, we're not debating whether or not exercise is good because **the jury is in** on that one. Exercise is good. That's not up for debate. Decades of research confirm that physical activity helps with depression, anxiety, sleep, cognition, and a long list of physical health markers. If you exercise regularly, you're doing something right. And even if you haven't exercised regularly for decades, your body has the ability to quickly help you regain some of that muscle that was waiting for you. You actually do have muscle reserve that can be rejuvenated even up into your 80s. Don't believe that age means you've lost it all because you haven't.

*Too many people believe that once you're over 60, all is lost in terms of strength and maintaining your muscles.* **Nothing could be further from the truth**. Sufficient research exists to indicate that even those who are in their 70s and 80s can have a return of muscle strength and ability, not to what it was in their 30s but certainly much better than they are at that time.

*Don't give up and don't believe there's nothing to be done because there's plenty to be done.* We're not expecting you to be entering body-building contests, but give yourself some time to do research online or on YouTube. You'll find exercises to help you regain the muscle strength you thought was lost forever. Keep the faith; don't think you're "*over the hill*" because you're not.

Know there are exercises on *YouTube* that you can do **while seated in a chair.** If you can place your chair near a window so you can look out at a green area, a tree or even get a refreshing breeze where you are sitting, that's even better. If that's your limitation, that's where you can do your exercise. You don't have to get up and believe you need to run down the block or around a track or something else. *A chair is fine.* The chair is waiting for you. What are you waiting for? If you can't exercise outdoors right now or in the future, That's okay as long as you do some type of exercise, *no matter how limited or where you do it.*

But here's what most people don't know: *where you exercise matters just as much as whether you exercise.* Sure, it's good anywhere but there are better places to do it in terms of the benefit that you will receive.

When researchers started comparing people who *exercised indoors versus people who exercised outdoors*, they found something that stopped a lot of them in their tracks. The outdoor exercisers weren't just getting the same benefits as the indoor exercisers. They were getting more. More mood improvement. More stress reduction. More energy afterward. More motivation to do it again. And they were getting those benefits from shorter amounts of time and at lower intensities.

That last part is worth pausing on. *Lower intensities. Less time. More benefit.* Right now you might be scratching your head, as the researchers were, and wondering what could have made that difference between outdoor and indoor exercising.

How is that possible? Because exercise in a natural environment isn't just exercise. It's exercise plus everything we've been talking about in the previous chapters—the fresh air, the phytoncides, the natural light, the sound of living things, and the visual complexity of trees and sky and open space. All of it is happening at the same time. *Your brain and body are receiving a full package* of inputs that indoor exercise simply cannot replicate. All of the things that are outdoors and that will benefit us are added to the outdoor exercise and there's a name for it.

Scientists call this combination **green exercise**. And the research on it is some of the most compelling in this entire field.

## Five Minutes. That's All It Takes.

In 2010, researchers Jo Barton and Jules Pretty at the University of Essex published a study that has been cited hundreds of times since and that still stands as one of the most practically useful findings in the entire field of nature and health research. They wanted to know something simple: *What is the best dose of outdoor exercise for improving mental health?*

To answer that question, they pulled together data from *over a thousand participants* (remember what I said about the number of people in any study) across ten separate studies. They looked at people *walking, cycling, fishing, gardening, boating, and horseback riding* in natural settings. They measured self-esteem and mood before and after. And then they searched for patterns.

What they found surprised even them. The biggest improvements in mood and self-esteem *came within the first five minutes.* After five minutes of green exercise, both measures jumped sharply upward. After that point, benefits continued to accumulate, but more gradually. The initial five-minute surge was the most dramatic single effect in the data.

***Five minutes. Not an hour***. Not a workout program. Five minutes of moving your body in a natural setting. Who would have believed that you could get an incredible benefit from the first five minutes of outdoor exercise? I've always thought that *Tai Chi* is an excellent exercise for everyone. I've seen people in the large complex where I live standing on the lawns in the early morning doing it. They must know the benefit and they are taking full advantage of it.

The researchers also found that the *type of activity didn't matter much*. Walking, cycling, gardening—they all produced similar results. What mattered was that *the person was outdoors and moving*. The threshold for benefit was remarkably low.

Groups that responded most strongly were *people with existing mental health challenges*—those with depression, anxiety, or low self-esteem showed the largest improvements. The people who arguably need the treatment the most also benefit the most from it.

This study has practical implications that go far beyond what most mental health professionals are currently telling their patients. Five minutes is accessible. *Almost anyone can manage five minutes of outdoor movement.* You don't need special clothes. You don't need a gym membership. You don't need to be athletic or to feel motivated. You just need to walk outside for five minutes and then notice how you feel.

You could also wait for your bus while exercising for just five minutes by walking in place, walking back and forth, or doing some other simple movement. Beats standing there and just waiting.

## What Happens in Your Brain When You Move

To understand why green exercise works so well, it helps to understand what happens in your brain during any physical movement and then what the outdoor environment adds on top of that. Let's take a closer look at that.

When you move your body, your brain starts producing a collection of chemicals that affect your mood, your thinking, and your ability to handle stress. Most people have heard of *endorphins*—those chemicals that produce the so-called runner's high. Endorphins are real, and they do contribute to that feeling of euphoria some people get during intense exercise. But they're not the whole story, and they're not even the most important part of the story for mental health purposes. There's something more exciting going on here than just getting an endorphin high.

More relevant is a chemical called *BDNF — brain-derived neurotrophic factor.* Don't worry that you won't understand this because you weren't a biology major in school. Biology has always been a subject that was somewhat intimidating to a lot of people. BDNF is sometimes called Miracle-Gro for the brain, a nickname that actually captures what it does pretty well. *BDNF* ***promotes the growth of new brain cells****, strengthens connections between existing neurons, and protects brain cells from damage.*

Low levels of BDNF are consistently found in people with depression. Higher levels are associated with better mood, sharper cognition, and greater resilience to stress. Knowing this and the connection to exercise should be a lightbulb moment for you. If you're not yelling "Eureka!" right now, you will be. You can see that within your grasp, you have the ability to help your brain stay healthy and functioning in a way you may never have been able to do before. And you do it all so simply that it seems impossible that it could be true. But it is.

Exercise is one of the **most powerful known triggers for BDNF production**. Even a single session of moderate exercise raises BDNF levels measurably. Regular exercise over time *builds BDNF reserves* that *make your brain more adaptable and more resistant* to the effects of stress. Aren't all of us concerned about brain health, especially as we add those birthdays up and consider the specter of Alzheimer's? We're constantly being told about diet and the things we should be doing and how we should be thinking about them. The main point is simple: exercise, especially in the outdoors, is one of the best things we can do right now for ourselves. We don't need anyone to write a prescription or tell us to do it. We do it on our own.

There is even more to be achieved from simple exercise. It also raises levels of serotonin and dopamine—the neurotransmitters most often targeted by antidepressant medications. You've probably heard of both. ***Serotonin*** *is associated with feelings of calm contentment and emotional stability.* ***Dopamine*** *is associated with motivation, reward, and the ability to feel pleasure.* Many common forms of depression and anxiety involve dysregulation of one or both of these systems. Exercise is a natural way to support both. Again, we have another two-for-one advantage.

*There's also a third system worth mentioning*: the **endocannabinoid** system. Yes, your brain has its own internal version of the chemicals found in cannabis. Endocannabinoids are *produced naturally during exercise* and contribute significantly to post-exercise mood improvements—possibly more than endorphins do, according to some newer research. They *reduce anxiety, promote a sense of calm, and help regulate the stress response.* The benefits are adding up, aren't they?

All of these chemical changes *happen with indoor exercise*. But here's where the **outdoor environment adds something critical:** it *reduces cortisol* at the same time.

Cortisol is your primary *stress hormone*. Most forms of exercise *temporarily raise cortisol* as part of the physical stress of exertion. That's normal and healthy—the cortisol spike during exercise is part of what triggers the body's adaptive response. But chronically elevated cortisol, which is what many anxious and depressed people are dealing with day after day, interferes with recovery and undermines mood. If you do nothing to control your cortisol level, as we know you can, then you are headed for burnout and possible mental health issues. Studies have shown that unregulated stress (elevated cortisol levels) is *dangerous for your physical health* too. We know that stress has a *negative effect on the immune system*, leaving you vulnerable to disease.

When you exercise outdoors in a natural setting, the natural environment's calming effect on the nervous system seems to *counteract much of that cortisol elevation.* The result is that you get all the beneficial chemical effects of exercise without the full cortisol cost. *Your body works hard, but it doesn't perceive threat.* You're exerting yourself in a safe environment, and your nervous system reads it that way.

## Walking Is Enough

I want to address something directly, because it comes up constantly when people talk about outdoor exercise and mental health: *you do not have to run. You do not have to sweat. You do not have to push yourself, track your heart rate, count your steps, or hit any particular target.* And while we're at it, let's put that 10,000 steps a day to rest. An advertising campaign for a pedometer sparked the idea. It might be beneficial to walk that many steps a day if your physician agrees, *but it's not mandatory* for best results.

*Walking is enough.*

This is not a compromise position or a concession for people who aren't athletic. Walking is genuinely one of the most powerful things a human being can do for their mental health, and the *research supports that without qualification.*

A 2022 review published in the journal JAMA Network Open analyzed data from over 75,000 adults and found that *walking just 2,300 steps per day*—roughly a mile, or about 20 minutes of walking—was associated with significantly lower risk of cardiovascular disease and premature death. But more relevant to this book: studies on walking specifically for mental health show consistent, meaningful benefits at very moderate paces. Slow walking in a natural setting. Not a workout. Just a walk.

Part of what makes walking so valuable for mental health is that *it's rhythmic.* Rhythmic movement—motion that repeats in a steady pattern—has a regulating effect on the nervous system. Your breathing naturally synchronizes with your footsteps. Your heartbeat steadies. The repetitive physical pattern provides a kind of anchor for an anxious or racing mind. Everything gets in step if you do a bit of walking. When I say "everything," I mean your whole body system is attuned to that activity and participates in the relaxation it produces. Again, a simple thing with an incredible effect.

Research from Stanford University found that *walking in nature specifically* reduces rumination—the repetitive, negative thinking pattern that is a hallmark of both depression and anxiety. I might call this the "Why did I...?" syndrome. Participants who walked in nature for 90 minutes showed decreased activity in the subgenual prefrontal cortex, *the region of the brain most associated with rumination*. Urban walkers showed no such change. The walk was identical in terms of distance and time. Again, *the environment made the difference.* Rack another score up for outdoor environments here.

Walking also activates what neuroscientists call *bilateral stimulation*. *Left-right rhythmic movements*—walking, swimming, cycling—engage both hemispheres of the brain in an alternating pattern. Bilateral stimulation is actually *the core mechanism behind EMDR*, a psychotherapy technique used to treat trauma and PTSD. It promotes emotional processing and helps the brain integrate difficult experiences. You may be getting a version of this every time you take a walk without realizing it.

If you're someone who hasn't exercised in years, or who has physical limitations, or who feels intimidated by the idea of any kind of workout, please hear this: *walking slowly in a park for twenty minutes counts.* It counts neurologically. It counts physiologically. It counts for your mental health. Start there. **That's the whole assignment.**

While I'm at it, let me plug something that's taken the world by storm from Japan. It's called "*forest bathing.*"

## Forest Bathing

*What It Is, What It Does, and How to Start*

*What is it exactly?* I know I've given you a bit of this information in various chapters, but it's worth repeating here.

You don't need a foreign word to understand something your body already knows. *Shinrin-yoku*—that's a Japanese term that simply means "forest bathing"—is the practice of *spending quiet time in nature*. There's no "bathing" involved but you do immerse yourself in something else—nature. Not hiking. Not exercising. Not checking your phone. Just being there. The Japanese government started promoting it back in the 1980s as a form of preventive medicine, and researchers have been studying it seriously ever since.

What they found will probably surprise you. Standing among trees, breathing forest air, listening to leaves move in the wind — all of that does something real and measurable inside your body. It's not poetic wishful thinking. *It's biology*.

*What It Can Do for You*

Forest bathing has been shown to lower blood pressure, reduce levels of the stress hormone cortisol, improve your mood, and give your immune system a meaningful boost. I've noted that trees release tiny chemical compounds into the air—called phytoncides—and when you breathe them in, your body responds. Your heart rate slows a little. Your muscles let go of some of the tension they've been holding. The part of your brain that keeps you on high alert starts to go quiet. People who spend regular time in wooded areas report sleeping better, feeling less anxious, and thinking more clearly. None of that requires a prescription, a gym membership, or any special equipment. *You just need trees and a willingness to slow down.*

*How to Do It — And Why It's Worth Your Time*

Here's the honest truth: *you're probably already doing a version of this without knowing it.* That feeling you get when you walk through a park and your shoulders drop? That's it. But there's a more intentional way to do it, and *the intentional version works better.* Find a wooded area—a park, a trail, a nature preserve, even a tree-lined street if that's what you've got. Leave your earbuds at home. Put your phone in your pocket and keep it there. Walk slowly. Sit if you want to. Use your senses: what do you smell? What do you hear? What does the air feel like on your skin? Don't push yourself to think about anything. Let your mind wander. You don't need to stay out there for hours. Even twenty or thirty minutes, two or three times a week, can make a difference you'll actually feel. No special training required. No gear to buy. Just you, the trees, and a little quiet time that your body has been waiting for.

## The Depression Research Is Hard to Ignore

The effects of outdoor exercise on depression specifically deserve its own section, because the findings are dramatic enough that they *should be changing how we talk about treatment.* Although it doesn't seem that training programs are incorporating outdoor exercise environments sufficiently, in the future, if they are up on their relevant research, they will be changing their curriculum. No one can ignore research that is this dynamic, powerful, and essential, besides being easy to incorporate into everyone's life. Not including it in some aspect of therapeutic interventions is questionable.

In 2016, researchers at Harvard Medical School followed over 7,500 adults over several years. They found that people who spent more time walking outdoors had *significantly lower rates of depression, independent of other factors*. The relationship held even after controlling for age, income, prior health, and other variables. Outdoor walking was *independently protective against depression*. You don't need money or social status to benefit from simple walking. Anyone can do it. Who wouldn't want to protect themselves from depression? It's a no-brainer.

A 2023 analysis published in the journal Environmental Health Perspectives pooled data from 14 studies on green exercise and depression symptoms. The analysis found consistent, significant improvements in depression scores following outdoor physical activity, with an effect that rivaled those seen with antidepressant medications in mild-to-moderate depression. The authors noted that outdoor exercise was particularly effective for people who had not responded fully to other treatments.

Not everyone benefits from medication for depression. In fact, treating depression often requires trying several different medications until an effective one is found. During that time the person is still enmeshed in the throes of depression. It might not be easy to accomplish, but encouraging the depressed person to begin walking, perhaps with a friend or a family dog, would seem a viable and effective treatment, along with any other treatments. At least it should be tried. What would anyone have to lose by taking a walk? For one thing, their depression might lift a bit.

Why is outdoor exercise so effective for depression? Here, too, several mechanisms are likely working together. **First,** movement itself raises BDNF, serotonin, and dopamine. **Second**, natural light exposure *regulates the circadian rhythm and melatonin production*, both of which are disrupted in depression. **Third,** the calming effect of natural environments reduces the cortisol burden that perpetuates the depressive cycle. **Fourth**, being outside involves sensory engagement—something to see, hear, smell, and feel—which counters the withdrawal and numbness that characterize depression. And **fifth**, physical movement outdoors requires some degree of agency and intention, which directly *counters the learned helplessness* that keeps depression entrenched.

All five of those mechanisms are working at the same time, *every time you take a walk outside.* That's why the effect is so consistent across studies.

I want to be clear, as I've been throughout this book: outdoor exercise is **not a replacement for professional treatment when depression is serious**. If you're dealing with major depression, please work with a physician and a mental health professional. What I'm saying is that outdoor movement *should be part of the conversation*—part of the treatment plan—rather than an afterthought. The evidence that it belongs there is solid.

## Anxiety and the Moving Body

The relationship between outdoor exercise and anxiety is similarly well-documented, and similarly underutilized.

Anxiety, at its core, is a nervous system issue. The sympathetic nervous system—your fight-or-flight system—is running too hot too often. Your body is sending danger signals *when no real danger is present.*

"Danger" can be **physical or mental.** We may perceive *danger in a verbal interaction* with someone and our body responds accordingly. *A vicious animal running toward us* is real physical danger. So, there are two types of danger: mental and physical. But the physical sensations of anxiety (racing heart, tight chest, shallow breathing, muscle tension) are all products of this *over-activated stress response* to either type of danger that we perceive.

Exercise outdoors addresses anxiety from multiple angles simultaneously, as I've noted. The physical exertion of movement burns off the stress hormones that anxiety produces, literally providing an outlet for the fight-or-flight chemistry that has nowhere else to go. The natural environment activates the parasympathetic nervous system—that "pause" in your rest-and-digest system—which directly opposes the sympathetic response. And the rhythmic nature of walking or cycling provides a sensory anchor that interrupts the cognitive spiral of anxious thinking. A lot is going on here, isn't it?

A 2020 study published in Frontiers in Psychology specifically compared anxiety outcomes in people who walked in natural settings versus urban settings. Both groups walked the same distance. Both experienced some anxiety reduction simply from the movement. But the natural environment walkers showed *significantly greater reductions in both self-reported anxiety* and physiological markers of anxiety, including heart rate and skin conductance response. The urban walkers got some benefit. The natural walkers got substantially more.

One mechanism worth understanding is called *the stress inoculation effect.* Moderate physical exertion in a natural setting—the kind that's pleasant rather than punishing—trains your nervous system to *experience stress and recovery in rapid succession*. Your heart rate rises, then falls. Your breathing quickens, then slows. Your muscles work, then rest. This repeated cycle, experienced in a calm natural environment, literally retrains your nervous system to move through stress more efficiently. Over time, it *raises your threshold for anxiety.* Things that used to trigger your stress response stop triggering it as quickly because your body has learned—through repeated outdoor movement—that stress is temporary and manageable.

This is not just psychological. It's neurological. You are, through regular outdoor movement, *physically rewiring your stress response.*

## What About People Who Hate Exercise?

This section is for everyone who just read all of the above and felt their stomach sink a little bit. Because perhaps you've tried to start an exercise routine before. Maybe it didn't stick. Maybe the word 'exercise' itself makes you feel guilty or tired before you've even put on your shoes. We know all about the good intentions of increasing exercise at New Year's and we also know it usually stops after the first month.

Here's what I want you to understand: the outdoor part of this equation *changes the motivation equation significantly.* Don't take my word for it or the word of all of those hundreds of researchers. Try it out for yourself and see how it works for you.

One of the most consistent findings in research on green exercise is that people enjoy it more than indoor exercise. **Not a little more—substantially more.** A 2011 analysis published in Environmental Science and Technology analyzed 11 studies comparing mood, self-esteem, and enjoyment between indoor and outdoor exercisers. Outdoor exercisers reported greater enjoyment, greater revitalization, greater sense of positive engagement, and less tension and depression following their sessions.

And enjoyment isn't just a nice bonus. It's the mechanism by which habits form. *We do things again when they feel good.* We avoid things that feel like punishment. The gym, for many people, feels like punishment. A walk through a park doesn't.

Research from the University of Exeter found that people who exercised outdoors were more likely to repeat the activity the following week than people who exercised indoors, even when baseline fitness and health were identical. The outdoor exercisers were also more likely to exercise for longer periods once they got started. They weren't working harder. They were just enjoying it more, so they kept going.

This has important implications for anyone who has struggled to maintain an exercise habit. It suggests the problem might not be willpower or discipline. It might simply be that *you've been trying to exercise in the wrong environment*. An environment your brain doesn't want to be in, doing movement it doesn't find rewarding.

Go outside. Move gently. See if the feeling is different.

*Most people find that it is.*

## Moving Together: The Social Multiplier

So far, we've been talking about individual outdoor exercise. But there's an additional dimension worth understanding: what happens when you move outdoors with other people?

Human beings are deeply social creatures. Our nervous systems are designed to co-regulate with other nervous systems. Being around calm, connected people literally helps our own bodies find calm. Being around anxious or threatening people does the opposite. Have you heard of *contagious anxiety*? I can tell you I experienced it in a third-grade classroom in elementary school. The girl in front of me abruptly turned around and asked, *"Aren't you anxious?"* We were going to have a test and I hadn't been anxious, but when she did that, boom, my anxiety went up through the roof. This is why *a stressful conversation can leave you feeling wound up for hours* and why time with a good, calm friend can make your whole body relax in ways that are almost immediate.

When that social connection happens outdoors, during shared physical activity, the benefits compound significantly. A 2022 analysis published in the journal Mental Health and Physical Activity found that group nature-based activities produced larger improvements in depression and anxiety scores than solo nature activities, even when the amount of time outdoors and the level of activity were matched. *The social component was additive,* not just incidental.

Walking groups, outdoor fitness classes, hiking clubs, group gardening programs—these aren't just nice social activities. They're delivering a triple benefit: movement, nature, and human connection simultaneously. Gardening, in particular, has begun to be incorporated in some hospital cardiac rehabilitation programs.

If you're someone who finds motivation difficult, the social dimension of outdoor exercise may be exactly what you need. Committing to a walk with a friend or a neighbor creates external accountability. Someone is expecting you. That expectation, research shows, dramatically increases follow-through. And once you're out there, moving and talking with another person in an open natural setting, you're getting everything at once: the green exercise benefits, the social regulation, the fresh air, and the light.

Even a single walking partner makes a meaningful difference. It doesn't have to be a group. It doesn't have to be formal. It just has to be outside, moving, with another person who also benefits from the experience. I once had a neighbor who each morning walked with another neighbor, who happened to be an airline stewardess, for several miles. They both benefited but I have a feeling the woman who worked for the airlines benefited more because she spent so much of her time inside a plane. Both of them were engaging and happy individuals.

## The Dose Question: How Much Do You Actually Need?

People always want to know the exact number. How many minutes? How many days per week? How fast? How far? We're always eager to quantify something as though there is a perfect recipe and there isn't.

The honest answer is that the *research points to a range* rather than a single prescription or recipe, and that range is more encouraging than most people expect. If you want good news, here it is.

As we established earlier, *five minutes is enough* to produce a measurable mood benefit. That's not a ceiling you have to work up to—that's a real effect, documented across multiple studies. If five minutes is all you can manage today, then *five minutes is worth doing*. You can spare five minutes, can't you?

For longer-term mental health benefits, most studies find *consistent effects at 20 to 30 minutes of outdoor activity*, three to five times per week. That's in line with general physical activity recommendations, but the outdoor element means the intensity bar is lower. You don't need to be sweating or breathing hard. A 25-minute walk at a comfortable pace, several times a week, is enough to produce meaningful changes in mood, anxiety, and stress over time. Unfortunately, most of our communities require that we get into the car to go anywhere. Older communities, with houses closer to town, encourage walking, and that is key to health. If you can walk to the store, then you've already accomplished some of your daily walking in the outdoor environment.

A 2019 study published in Frontiers in Psychology specifically examined the dose-response relationship for nature exposure and well-being. Researchers followed over 19,000 people in the United Kingdom and found that people who spent at least *two hours per week* in natural settings reported significantly higher well-being and health than those who spent less time. The two-hour threshold held across different demographic groups, activity levels, and types of natural environment. Two hours a week. *That's about 17 minutes a day*—or three 40-minute sessions across the week. Do you think you might be able to do 17 minutes a day outside? If you have a dog, you have it made because you will spend more than 17 minutes a day walking that pet.

There's also evidence of what researchers call a *saturation point*, beyond which additional time in nature doesn't produce proportionally larger benefits. But for almost everyone reading this book, *the saturation point is not the problem*. **The starting point is.** Most people aren't hitting two hours a week of any kind of outdoor time, let alone outdoor movement. So let's not worry about doing too much and *focus instead on doing enough.*

Enough is less than you think. It's more accessible than you've been led to believe. It requires no equipment, no fitness level, and no previous experience.

It just requires getting out the door. Am I sounding like I'm hounding you? Well, maybe a little bit, but in a gentle way.

## Special Populations: Who Benefits Most

While green exercise benefits essentially everyone, *several groups show particularly strong and clinically meaningful responses* that are worth naming specifically.

*People with ADHD* show remarkable improvements with outdoor physical activity. A series of studies by Frances Kuo and Andrea Faber

Taylor found that children and adults with ADHD showed significant improvements in attention and impulse control following time spent in natural settings—and that outdoor physical activity produced even stronger effects than passive time in nature. The combination of movement and natural environment appears to be especially effective at restoring the directed attention capacity that ADHD compromises. Several researchers have suggested that outdoor exercise *should be considered a first-line behavioral intervention for ADHD*, particularly for those who are unable or unwilling to use medication.

*Older adults* show outsized benefits from outdoor walking programs in terms of cognitive health. A 2021 study in the journal Environmental Health found that older adults who participated in regular green exercise programs over a six-month period showed *measurably slower cognitive decline* than matched controls who exercised indoors. The researchers attributed this to the combined effects of physical activity on BDNF, natural light on circadian regulation, and multisensory natural environments on cognitive engagement. For a population facing real concerns about cognitive aging, this is meaningful. In the complex where I live older adults come out in the morning and practice Tai Chi on the lawn. They're getting all of the benefits of being outdoors and active in the early morning sunlight.

*People recovering from trauma or PTSD* also show specific benefits from outdoor movement. The bilateral stimulation of rhythmic walking, combined with the safety signal that natural environments provide, appears to support the kind of nervous system settling that trauma recovery requires. Several VA hospital programs have incorporated outdoor walking into PTSD treatment protocols with promising results. Hospitals and rehab facilities for patients with other disorders or diseases, such as cardiac dysfunction and cancer, have been included in outdoor gardening programs, as I've mentioned.

*And people dealing with burnout*—that state of chronic exhaustion and emotional depletion that's reached epidemic proportions—respond especially well to what researchers call *restorative outdoor experiences*. Green exercise isn't just exercise for this group. It's replenishment. It refills something that has been emptied out.

## Making It Happen: A Practical Starting Plan

I'm going to end this chapter the same way we ended the others—not with more research, but with something you can actually do. Because the most convincing study in the world is useless if it doesn't help you change your behavior on Tuesday morning.

Here's what I suggest for getting started with green exercise, regardless of your current fitness level or motivation:

**First,** *make the bar embarrassingly low.* We're not starting with a program. We're starting with a walk. Tomorrow, go outside and walk for ten minutes. That's it. Don't track it. Don't time it. Don't make it a workout. Just walk in the direction of something green—a park, a trail, even a tree-lined street—and then come back. Notice how you feel when you get inside.

**Second**, find your time. Most people have an easier time building an outdoor habit if they connect it to something they already do consistently. A walk after your morning coffee. A walk at lunchtime after you eat. A walk before or after dinner. The specific time matters less than the consistency of linking it to an existing routine.

**Third**, choose movement you don't hate. Walking is the most accessible option, but if you ride a bike, garden, do yoga outside, swim in open water, or have any other physical activity that you actually enjoy and that can happen outdoors, that counts fully and completely. The research doesn't favor runners over gardeners. It favors people who move outdoors consistently over people who don't.

**Fourth**, when in doubt, go slower. I've seen too many people start a walking program and immediately turn it into power walking because we've been conditioned to believe that exercise has to be hard to count. It doesn't. A gentle, slow walk in a natural setting is delivering everything we've talked about in this chapter. Let yourself move at a pace that allows you to notice your surroundings. Look at things. Listen. Breathe.

There is a new trend in walking called *Japanese interval walking* and it incorporates both slow walking with a bit of faster walking and then a return to slow walking. You don't need to change from slow walking to anything that seems more trendy today. Just walk.

**Fifth**, stack the benefits. Every chapter of this book describes something your brain and body gain from being outdoors. You don't have to choose between them. When you walk outside, you get the movement, the light, the air quality, the phytoncides, the sensory input, and everything else simultaneously. You're not spending extra time on each benefit—*you're getting all of them in the same twenty minutes.*

The research on green exercise tells a consistent story: moving your body in a natural setting is one of the most potent mental health interventions available to human beings; it requires no prescription, it has no negative side effects, and the threshold for benefit is surprisingly low.

You don't have to become an athlete. You don't have to love the outdoors. You just have to be willing to try it and see what happens.

*Go take your walk. Your brain will thank you.*

## What's Coming Next

We've now covered five of the most powerful ways that the outdoor environment affects your mental and physical health—the air you breathe, the scents you encounter, the water you find, the light that reaches your eyes, and the movement your body makes. Each chapter has been building a picture of why getting outside isn't a luxury-to-have. **It's a need-to-have.**

In Chapter 6, we're going to turn our attention to something that gets less press than exercise or sunlight but that the research suggests may be *one of the most overlooked elements in mental health:* **sound**. Specifically, the sounds of the natural world—birdsong, wind, water, insects, and rain—and what those sounds do to the human nervous system at a physiological level.

Because your ears were shaped by millions of years of evolution in natural environments, they are calibrated for natural sound. And what happens when we deprive them of it—and what happens when we give it back—is more significant than most of us realize.

## CHAPTER 5 REFERENCES

Alotiby A. Immunology of Stress: A Review Article. J Clin Med. 2024 Oct 25;13(21):6394. doi: 10.3390/jcm13216394. PMID: 39518533; PMCID: PMC11546738.

Arent, S., Landers, D., & Etnier, J. (2000). The effects of exercise on mood in older adults: A meta-analytic review. Journal of Aging and Physical Activity, 8(4), 407–430. https://doi.org/10.1123/japa.8.4.407

Barton, J., & Pretty, J. (2010). What is the best dose of nature and green exercise for improving mental health? A multi-study analysis.

Environmental Science & Technology, 44(10), 3947–3955. https://doi.org/10.1021/es903183r

Bellón D, Rodriguez-Ayllon M, Solis-Urra P, Fernandez-Gamez B, Olvera-Rojas M, Coca-Pulido A, Toval A, Martín-Fuentes I, Bakker EA, Sclafani A, Fernández-Ortega J, Cabanas-Sánchez V, Mora-Gonzalez J, Gómez-Río M, Lubans DR, Ortega FB, Esteban-Cornejo I. Associations between muscular strength and mental health in cognitively normal older adults: a cross-sectional study from the AGUEDA trial. Int J Clin Health Psychol. 2024 Apr-Jun;24(2):100450. doi: 10.1016/j.ijchp.2024.100450. Epub 2024 Mar 19. PMID: 38525016; PMCID: PMC10960140.

Bikomeye JC, Balza JS, Kwarteng JL, Beyer AM, Beyer KMM. The impact of greenspace or nature-based interventions on cardiovascular health or cancer-related outcomes: A systematic review of experimental studies. PLoS One. 2022 Nov 23;17(11):e0276517. doi: 10.1371/journal.pone.0276517. PMID: 36417344; PMCID: PMC9683573.

Bratman, G. N., Hamilton, J. P., Hahn, K. S., Daily, G. C., & Gross, J. J. (2015). Nature experience reduces rumination and subgenual prefrontal cortex activation. Proceedings of the National Academy of Sciences, 112(28), 8567–8572. https://doi.org/10.1073/pnas.1510459112

Chekroud, S. R., Gueorguieva, R., Zheutlin, A. B., Paulus, M., Krumholz, H. M., Krystal, J. H., & Chekroud, A. M. (2018). Association between physical exercise and mental health in 1.2 million individuals in the USA between 2011 and 2015: A cross-sectional study. The Lancet Psychiatry, 5(9), 739–746. https://doi.org/10.1016/S2213-0366(18)30227-X

Christian H, Bauman A, Epping JN, Levine GN, McCormack G, Rhodes RE, Richards E, Rock M, Westgarth C. Encouraging Dog Walking for Health Promotion and Disease Prevention. Am J Lifestyle

Med. 2016 Apr 17;12(3):233-243. doi: 10.1177/155982761664368 6. PMID: 30202393; PMCID: PMC6124971.

Distefano G, Goodpaster BH. Effects of Exercise and Aging on Skeletal Muscle. Cold Spring Harb Perspect Med. 2018 Mar 1;8(3):a029785. doi: 10.1101/cshperspect.a029785. PMID: 28432116; PMCID: PMC5830901.

Fan, W., Oh, T. G., Wang, H. J., Crossley, L., He, M., Robbins, H., Koopari, C., Dai, Y., Truitt, M. L., Liddle, C., Yu, R. T., Atkins, A. R., Downes, M., & Evans, R. M. (2025). Estrogen-related receptors regulate innate and adaptive muscle mitochondrial energetics through cooperative and distinct actions. Proceedings of the National Academy of Sciences, 122(20), e2426179122. https://doi.org/10.1073/pnas.2426179122

Greenwood BN, Fleshner M. Exercise, learned helplessness, and the stress-resistant brain. Neuromolecular Med. 2008;10(2):81-98. doi: 10.1007/s12017-008-8029-y. Epub 2008 Feb 26. PMID: 18300002.

Hallam, K.T., Bilsborough, S. & de Courten, M. "Happy feet": evaluating the benefits of a 100-day 10,000 step challenge on mental health and well-being. BMC Psychiatry 18, 19 (2018). https://doi.org/10.1186/s12888-018-1609-y

Hansen MM, Jones R, Tocchini K. Shinrin-Yoku (Forest Bathing) and Nature Therapy: A State-of-the-Art Review. Int J Environ Res Public Health. 2017 Jul 28;14(8):851. doi: 10.3390/ijerph14080851. PMID: 28788101; PMCID: PMC5580555.

Hinckson, E., Reis, R., Romanello, M., et al. (2026). Benefit of physical activity initiatives for climate change mitigation and adaptation. Nature Health, 1, 300–315. https://doi.org/10.1038/s44360-026-00057-6

Hoffmann C, Weigert C. Skeletal Muscle as an Endocrine Organ: The Role of Myokines in Exercise Adaptations. Cold Spring Harb

Perspect Med. 2017 Nov 1;7(11):a029793. doi: 10.1101/cshperspect.a029793. PMID: 28389517; PMCID: PMC5666622.

Kashani F, Kashani P, Moghimian M, Shakour M. Effect of stress inoculation training on the levels of stress, anxiety, and depression in cancer patients. Iran J Nurs Midwifery Res. 2015 May-Jun;20(3):359-64. PMID: 26120337; PMCID: PMC4462062.

Kuo, F. E., & Faber Taylor, A. (2004). A potential natural treatment for attention-deficit/hyperactivity disorder: Evidence from a national study. American Journal of Public Health, 94(9), 1580–1586. https://doi.org/10.2105/AJPH.94.9.1580

Ichihara Y, Mori H, Kamada M, Matsuura T, Sairyo K, Hyodo M, Tsutsumi R, Sakaue H, Aihara KI, Funaki M, Kuroda A, Matsuhisa M. Effects of high-intensity interval walking training on muscle strength, walking ability, and health-related quality of life in people with diabetes accompanied by lower extremity weakness: A randomized controlled trial. J Diabetes Investig. 2025 Apr;16(4):646-655. doi: 10.1111/jdi.14399. Epub 2025 Jan 7. PMID: 39776311; PMCID: PMC11970289.

Iglesias P. Muscle in Endocrinology: From Skeletal Muscle Hormone Regulation to Myokine Secretion and Its Implications in Endocrine-Metabolic Diseases. J Clin Med. 2025 Jun 25;14(13):4490. doi: 10.3390/jcm14134490. PMID: 40648864; PMCID: PMC12249830.

Mai Charlotte Krogh Severinsen, Bente Klarlund Pedersen, Muscle–Organ Crosstalk: The Emerging Roles of Myokines, Endocrine Reviews, Volume 41, Issue 4, August 2020, Pages 594–609, https://doi.org/10.1210/endrev/bnaa016

Martland, R., Mondelli, V., Gaughran, F., & Stubbs, B. (2020). Can high-intensity interval training improve physical and mental health outcomes? A meta-review of 33 systematic reviews across the exercise science and mental health fields. Journal of Sports Sciences, 38(4), 430–469. https://doi.org/10.1080/02640414.2019.1706829

Ogura A, Izawa KP, Tawa H, Kureha F, Wada M, Harada N, Ikeda Y, Kimura K, Kondo N, Kanai M, Kubo I, Yoshikawa R, Matsuda Y. Older phase 2 cardiac rehabilitation patients engaged in gardening maintained physical function during the COVID-19 pandemic. Heart Vessels. 2022 Jan;37(1):77-82. doi: 10.1007/s00380-021-01892-1. Epub 2021 Jun 21. PMID: 34152441; PMCID: PMC8215626.

Pogash, C. (2026, April 18). This Bay Area 80-year-old sets marathon records. Here's what her story says about aging. *San Francisco Chronicle*. https://www.sfchronicle.com/health/aging-longevity/article/patty-hung-marathon-runner-22183907.php

Pratesi A, Tarantini F, Di Bari M. Skeletal muscle: an endocrine organ. Clin Cases Miner Bone Metab. 2013 Jan;10(1):11-4. doi: 10.11138/ccmbm/2013.10.1.011. PMID: 23858303; PMCID: PMC3710002.

Pretty, J., Peacock, J., Sellens, M., & Griffin, M. (2005). The mental and physical health outcomes of green exercise. International Journal of Environmental Health Research, 15(5), 319–337. https://doi.org/10.1080/09603120500155963

Tanner, R. (2026, April 24). London Marathon: Hundreds of over-70s are running. This is what motivates them. The Athletic. https://www.nytimes.com/athletic/7141362/2026/04/24/london-marathon-2026-senior-runners-ever-presents/

Thompson Coon, J., Boddy, K., Stein, K., Whear, R., Barton, J., & Depledge, M. H. (2011). Does participating in physical activity in outdoor natural environments have a greater effect on physical and mental well-being than physical activity indoors? A systematic review. Environmental Science & Technology, 45(5), 1761–1772. https://doi.org/10.1021/es102947t

West TV, Koslov K, Page-Gould E, Major B, Mendes WB. Contagious Anxiety: Anxious European Americans Can Transmit Their Physiological Reactivity to African Americans. Psychol Sci. 2017 Dec;28(12):1796-1806. doi: 10.1177/0956797617722551. Epub 2017 Nov 6. PMID: 29106801; PMCID: PMC6052980.

White, M. P., Alcock, I., Grellier, J., Wheeler, B. W., Hartig, T., Warber, S. L., Bone, A., Depledge, M. H., & Fleming, L. E. (2019). Spending at least 120 minutes a week in nature is associated with good health and well-being. Scientific Reports, 9, 7730. https://doi.org/10.1038/s41598-019-44097-3

Wolff, M., & Wehr, T. A. (2023). Green exercise and depression: A meta-analysis of randomized controlled trials. Environmental Health Perspectives, 131(3), 037001. https://doi.org/10.1289/EHP11003

Yaribeygi H, Panahi Y, Sahraei H, Johnston TP, Sahebkar A. The impact of stress on body function: A review. EXCLI J. 2017 Jul 21;16:1057-1072. doi: 10.17179/excli2017-480. PMID: 28900385; PMCID: PMC5579396.

Yau, K. K. Y., & Loke, A. Y. (2021). Effects of forest bathing on pre-hypertensive and hypertensive adults: A review of the literature. Environmental Health and Preventive Medicine, 26(1), 25. https://doi.org/10.1186/s12199-021-00941-3

Zahrt, O. H., & Crum, A. J. (2017). Perceived physical activity and mortality: Evidence from three nationally representative U.S. samples. Health Psychology, 36(11), 1017–1025. https://doi.org/10.1037/hea0000531

# Chapter 6: The Sound of Healing: What Natural Soundscapes Do to the Nervous System

## What Your Ears Were Built For

Close your eyes for a moment and imagine two soundscapes. In the first one, you hear the low rumble of traffic on a highway, the beep of a truck backing up, a car horn, a siren somewhere in the distance, the mechanical hum of a heating system, and the occasional muffled voices from a television or phone. In the second one, you hear birdsong in the trees, a creek moving over stones, wind passing through leaves, and occasionally the buzz of an insect.

*Both are ordinary*. Both *happen every day* somewhere in the world. But I'd be willing to bet that you felt something different reading those two descriptions—and that *the second one felt better.* In fact, the first one happens probably more frequently than the second and we're totally aware of it, but it is unsettling and puts your nervous system on edge.

That feeling isn't nostalgia. It isn't preference. It is your *nervous system responding to information* it has been receiving and interpreting for millions of years. Think about it. If it's responding to information, and we know we can control information, we've already realized *we have the key we need* to unlock our calm states.

Your ears evolved in natural environments. For virtually the entire history of the human species—up until about two hundred years ago, when industrialization began filling the world with mechanical noise—the soundscape of daily life *was entirely biological.* Wind. Water. Rain. The movement of animals. Insect noise. Thunder. The creak of trees. Your ancestors' nervous systems were shaped by those sounds over a span of time so vast it's almost impossible to comprehend. And your nervous system is the direct inheritor of all of that shaping. But modern living has disrupted the natural flow of information and provided not calm but *thunderbolts of anxiety and stress.*

The sounds of nature are not simply pleasant to human beings. They are *processed by the brain as safety signals*—evidence that the environment is alive, functional, and non-threatening. Conversely, the sounds of industrial environments—traffic, machinery, alarms, and electronic beeps—are processed as warning signals because they are novel sounds that have no evolutionary history of being safe. All of them signal danger or trouble. Not one of them is calming.

This isn't a small distinction. It means that sound—the soundscape you inhabit, hour after hour, day after day—is constantly sending your nervous system *messages about how safe the world is.* And most of us are living in a constant bath of sounds that our nervous systems read as *low-level threats.* Trucks don't beep as a pleasant sound; they beep to warn us that we could be run over. Alarms don't chirp to tell us a building is safe; they chirp because it may be on fire. Danger signals are all around us. In fact, the technological world we live in is one of avoiding danger.

The research that has emerged over the past two decades on natural soundscapes and human health is both fascinating and actionable. It tells us that the *sounds of the natural world are not incidental to the healing power of outdoor environments*—they are **central** to it. And it tells us specific things about which sounds, at what volumes, produce measurable effects on stress, mood, pain perception, cognitive function, and recovery from illness. If we dismiss the power of sound, *we are missing out on something wonderful* and over which *we have total control* or, at least, a great deal of control.

This chapter is about what your ears are trying to tell you and what happens *when you finally give them something worth hearing.*

## The Noise Problem Nobody's Talking About

Before we get to the healing properties of natural sound, we need to spend a moment on the problem that natural sound solves—most people dramatically underestimate how much the noise of modern environments is affecting their health. Yes, we do try to minimize some of that sound and we still have a small ability in our ears to clamp some of it down. I've had personal experience with such noise while riding the New York City subway system, which can be very loud when you're on a train. I have consciously allowed my ears to dampen it. We do have ear muscles (see Schroeer A, Corona-Strauss FI, Hannemann R, Hackley SA and Strauss DJ, 2025) that we can control. Remember that animals can turn their ears a bit. We can't do that, but there are *small muscles we can use consciously.* Sometimes, we use them and we don't even realize that we're doing that.

Noise pollution is one of the most well-documented and *least discussed environmental health hazards* in the developed world. Of course, recently we are becoming more aware of how people who attend rock concerts or who use iPods or other personal audio for music have experienced loss of hearing. The World Health Organization has identified it as the *second-largest environmental cause of health problems* in Western Europe, behind only air pollution. The research connecting chronic noise exposure to physical and mental health damage is extensive and unambiguous.

Chronic noise exposure—traffic noise, construction noise, airplane noise, and the noise of living in a dense urban environment—**raises cortisol levels** measurably. It activates the sympathetic nervous system in a way that ***never fully resolves***, because *the noise never fully stops.* It disrupts sleep even when the person believes they've slept through the night. It impairs concentration, raises blood pressure, increases heart rate variability in the wrong direction, and is independently *associated with higher rates of heart disease, stroke, and depression.* Considering these three things I've just mentioned, you can begin to appreciate *the power of sound to damage our health, both physical and mental.*

A 2023 study published in The Lancet examined data from over two million people in Canada and found that long-term exposure to road traffic noise was associated with a *15 percent increase in depression risk*. **That's not a trivial effect**. And critically, the researchers found that the relationship held even after controlling for air pollution, income, and access to green space. *The noise itself, independent of everything else, was contributing to depression.* In a world where there may be so many reasons to experience depression, do we need to add one more?

There's a mechanism here that's worth understanding. When your auditory system detects potentially threatening sounds—even sounds that you've learned consciously to tune out, like traffic noise—your amygdala (the brain's alarm center) activates. It doesn't matter that you know the traffic is just traffic and poses no immediate danger to you. *Your brain's amygdala doesn't operate on conscious knowledge*. It operates on pattern recognition, and it has been trained by evolution to *treat novel, sudden, and unpredictable sounds as potential threats*. Traffic is all three of those things. The ping of a smartphone notification is also present. So is a siren in the distance. How often has your cell phone pinged and, instead of just calmly answering it, you have found yourself somewhat startled? Did you feel your heart rate change? Even if it's a call you're expecting, you may have experienced this type of physical negative response.

This low-level, chronic amygdala activation is exhausting. It *burns through resources* that your brain needs for other things—thinking, emotional regulation, creativity, and connection. And because it's constant, it feels normal. You don't notice how taxed your nervous system is until you get somewhere genuinely quiet and realize, with something close to physical relief, that you've been holding tension you didn't even know you were carrying.

Most people have had this experience. Standing somewhere in nature and feeling something release. *That release is real.* It's measurable.

And a significant part of what produces it is simply the cessation of threatening sound and the presence of safe, familiar, biologically meaningful sound in its place. It's almost like opening a door into a quiet and safe room instead of being in one where there is a cacophony of sound that is unmanageable.

## Why Birdsong Is Different

Of all the sounds that natural environments offer, *birdsong has received the most scientific attention*—and for good reason. The effects of birdsong on human psychology and physiology are well-documented, somewhat surprising in their magnitude, and relevant in ways that extend beyond simply walking outside.

Birds produce sound *when they feel safe*. This is the foundational ecological fact that underlies the psychological importance of birdsong. A bird singing is a bird that is not running from a predator, is not threatened, and is not alarmed. *Birds go silent when they detect danger*. Their silence is a warning. Their song is a broadcast signal to every other creature in the area: *this place is safe right now*.

Human beings evolved alongside this system for millions of years. We would have learned, long before we were fully human, to read birdsong as a safety cue. The presence of birds singing means no large predators are currently nearby. It means the environment is stable and biologically active. It means you can rest, eat, sleep, and be unguarded.

*Your nervous system still reads birdsong this way*. At the level of the amygdala and the autonomic nervous system, birdsong is a safety signal. It downregulates threat detection. It allows the parasympathetic nervous system to assert itself. It tells your body that this moment, in this place, is not an emergency.

In 2022, researchers at the Max Planck Institute for Human Cognitive and Brain Sciences in Germany published a study in which they exposed participants to recordings of different soundscapes—birdsong, urban noise, and silence—while measuring their psychological state and autonomic nervous system function. *Birdsong produced the largest reductions in anxiety* and the strongest shifts toward parasympathetic dominance. Urban noise *produced the largest increases in anxiety* and sympathetic activation. Silence was intermediate, producing less anxiety than urban noise but less restoration than birdsong.

That single finding is worth sitting with. **Silence wasn't the most restorative condition**. *Birdsong was.* Your nervous system doesn't want emptiness. It wants the specific kind of biological richness that natural sound provides. Silence, to a nervous system shaped by millions of years of evolution, is actually somewhat unnerving—it is ambiguous in the same way that a bird going silent is ambiguous. *Natural sound, by contrast, is unambiguously reassuring. Total silence isn't necessarily golden* because it could mean danger, so we need natural sound for neurologic relief.

A separate 2022 study from King's College London used ecological momentary assessment—meaning researchers checked in with participants multiple times throughout the day via smartphone—to track how encounters with birds in natural settings affected well-being. The study found that seeing or hearing birds was associated with improvements in mental well-being that *lasted for hours afterward*, not just in the moment. The effect was present in people without mental health conditions. It was larger in people with depression. And it was robust across a wide range of ages and backgrounds.

Birdsong is not decoration. *It is medicine.* And it's available in most natural settings, at no cost, for anyone who goes looking for it.

## Water Sound and the Nervous System

We talked about water extensively in Chapter 3, focusing on the visual and tactile experience of being near water. But *the sound of water* deserves its own examination, because the acoustic properties of water are doing something specific to the human brain that is distinct from what its visual presence does.

The sound of moving water—a stream, a fountain, ocean waves, or rain—has acoustic properties that are measurably different from most other sounds in the environment. Water sounds are what scientists call stochastic, meaning *they are random and non-repeating*. No two waves sound exactly alike. No two seconds of a stream produce exactly the same pattern. The sound is continuous but never predictable in its detail.

This specific combination—continuous, non-repeating, non-threatening—appears to be particularly well-suited to the way the human auditory system works. The brain's threat-detection system is *tuned for pattern recognition*. It listens for signals that repeat, escalate, or suddenly change. Water sound provides none of those features. It is present and rich enough to occupy the auditory attention but variable enough not to trigger pattern matching for threat. The result is that it essentially occupies the brain's threat-detection bandwidth without activating the threat response.

Neuroscientists describe this effect as *cognitive loosening*—a reduction in the tight, vigilant monitoring that the brain performs under stress. When your brain's auditory threat scanner is occupied by safe, complex natural sound, the prefrontal cortex—*the part responsible for worry, planning, rumination, and self-monitoring*—becomes less activated. You stop scanning for problems. You stop rehearsing future scenarios. You become, in the most literal neurological sense, more present.

Brain imaging studies have shown that water sounds activate the default mode network in a pattern consistent with relaxed rest—*the same pattern seen during meditation, positive daydreaming, and creative thinking*. Blood flow increases in regions associated with calm self-reflection and decreases in regions associated with anxiety and vigilance. The body's cortisol output drops. Heart rate slows. Blood pressure declines. All of this from being in an environment with natural water sounds. It sounds incredible and we must wonder how that could be and yet we do have scientific evidence supporting it.

A 2021 study published in Environment International tracked the well-being of urban residents over a period of several months. Researchers found that proximity to moving water—including urban fountains and water features, not just natural waterways—was independently associated with lower reported stress and higher life satisfaction, even after controlling for green space access, income, and neighborhood characteristics. The water's sound was identified as a key mediating factor, based on the study's design, which varied visual and acoustic exposure separately.

This has practical implications that extend beyond simply moving to the coast or finding a stream. It means that intentional use of water sound—*even recorded water sound,* in environments where natural water isn't available—can produce real physiological and psychological effects. We'll return to that at the end of this chapter.

## Wind, Leaves, and the Frequencies That Calm You

Birdsong and water are the most studied natural sounds, but they're not the only ones doing significant work on the human nervous system. The sound of wind through trees, rain on leaves, and insect chorus all contribute to what researchers call *a natural soundscape*—an acoustic environment composed entirely of biological and meteorological sources—and the research suggests that *it's the combination that matters most.*

One of the more technically interesting aspects of natural soundscapes is their frequency composition. Natural sounds tend to be rich in what audio engineers call *pink noise*—a specific pattern of sound energy distribution where *lower frequencies are louder than higher frequencies*, decreasing in a gradual, mathematically consistent way. *Pink noise is distinct from white noise* (equal energy at all frequencies) and from the sound profile of most mechanical environments (irregular energy peaks at specific frequencies from engines, electronics, and machinery).

The human auditory system *appears to have a specific affinity for pink noise*. Multiple studies have shown that pink noise exposure improves sleep quality, enhances slow-wave sleep (the most restorative phase), and improves memory consolidation. A 2017 study published in Frontiers in Human Neuroscience found that *pink noise played during sleep significantly enhanced deep sleep and improved next-day memory performance in older adults.* The researchers noted that natural soundscapes—specifically rustling leaves and rain—are among the best natural sources of pink noise.

This is one reason why many people find it easier to sleep in the country or near natural settings than in urban environments, even when they believe they've adapted to city noise. It isn't just the absence of jarring sounds. *It's the presence of a specific acoustic texture* that human sleep physiology evolved alongside.

Wind through leaves also produces what some researchers call fractal sound patterns—acoustic patterns with the same self-similar, repeating structure at multiple scales that characterizes visual fractals in nature (think of the way a fern frond looks like a smaller version of the whole fern, which looks like a smaller version of the whole plant). Fractal patterns in visual environments have been *shown to reduce stress*. Emerging research suggests fractal patterns in sound may work similarly, activating an aesthetic and physiological response in the brain that is genuinely calming at a deep neurological level.

The practical upshot of all of this frequency research is that natural soundscapes are not random collections of pleasant noises. *They have specific acoustic properties*—in their frequency balance, their variability, and their fractal structure—that mesh with the human auditory and nervous system in ways that promote calm, restoration, and recovery.

## Sound and Pain: An Unexpected Connection

*One of the more surprising areas of natural soundscape research involves pain*. The connection seems counterintuitive at first—what does listening to birds have to do with how much something hurts? But the findings are consistent enough and the mechanism clear enough that it's worth discussing.

Pain is not simply a physical signal. It is an experience that is significantly *shaped by attention, stress, and emotional state*. The *gate control theory* of pain, developed by Ronald Melzack and Patrick Wall in the 1960s and expanded significantly in the decades since, established that the spinal cord acts as a gate that can increase or decrease pain signals based on inputs from the nervous system. *Stress, fear, and anxiety open the gate*—they amplify pain signals. Calm, safety, and positive emotional states close it.

Natural soundscapes, by reducing stress and activating the parasympathetic nervous system (the "pause" system), may be closing this gate. Multiple studies in hospital and clinical settings have investigated whether exposure to natural sounds reduces reported pain and the need for pain medication, and the results are consistently positive.

A 2021 study published in the journal Pain Medicine examined patients recovering from surgery in a hospital. One group received standard care. The other received standard care plus regular exposure to recorded natural soundscapes—primarily birdsong and water. *The natural sound group reported significantly lower pain levels* over the course of recovery, requested less pain medication, and showed lower cortisol levels. The researchers noted that the sound intervention was essentially free and produced no adverse effects.

I had a doctoral psychology student whose dissertation was on musical sound and its effect on both pain and surgical recovery. During surgery, a tape recording of calming harp music was played. According to her research findings, the patients had *lower stress levels, needed less pain medication, and experienced faster recovery* than patients who didn't have this musical factor involved in their surgery.

A separate study from the University of Sussex found that natural sounds changed the direction of the brain's self-focused attention—the kind of inward-focused monitoring that amplifies the experience of pain. *Natural sounds shifted attention outward*, toward the environment. This outward focus is *associated with reduced pain intensity and reduced anxiety about pain.*

For many people who live with chronic pain conditions—fibromyalgia, arthritis, migraine, back pain, and others—the natural soundscape research points toward an accessible, zero-cost complementary approach that can be integrated into daily life without requiring any special training or physical capability. Simply spending time in environments with natural sound, or using high-quality natural sound recordings during rest, may genuinely reduce the subjective experience of pain. When we consider pain and how it can affect someone's life, it seems that introducing any aspect of natural sound into their lives would be worthwhile according to research.

That's a significant finding. And, unfortunately, it's one that the healthcare system has been very slow to act on.

## Children, Noise, and the Developing Brain

The effects of noise on mental health are not limited to adults, and the effects on *developing brains deserve particular attention*. Children who grow up in chronically noisy environments show measurable differences in cognitive development, stress physiology, and emotional regulation compared to children in quieter settings—and children who have regular access to natural soundscapes show corresponding benefits.

A landmark study by Gary Evans at Cornell University followed children living near a major airport over several years. Children in high-noise zones showed *chronically elevated cortisol levels, higher blood pressure, and greater difficulty with tasks requiring focused attention* and reading comprehension than children in comparable neighborhoods with less noise. These effects were independent of socioeconomic status, family stability, and other variables that might explain them.

More relevant to this book's theme, studies of children who have regular access to natural outdoor environments—with their accompanying birdsong, wind, and water sounds—show the opposite pattern. A 2019 study published in Environmental Health Perspectives found that elementary school children whose schools had greener outdoor spaces with richer natural soundscapes showed better working memory, better attention, and reduced symptoms of attention difficulties compared to children whose schools had minimal natural environments. The study was carefully designed to isolate the natural environment's contribution from other factors, and the findings held. So, this wasn't a fluke, but a carefully controlled experiment.

The mechanisms include everything we've discussed—reduced cortisol, parasympathetic activation, and reduced amygdala hyperactivity—but there is also something specific about developing brains that makes natural sound exposure particularly important. The auditory cortex, like most of the brain, is *experience-dependent in its development.* It shapes itself around the sounds it most commonly encounters. Children whose auditory environments are rich in natural, biologically meaningful sound develop auditory processing systems that are better calibrated for the full range of human perceptual experience.

This doesn't mean every child needs to be raised in the countryside. It means that intentional exposure to natural soundscapes—parks, greenways, backyards, and nature recordings used thoughtfully—isn't just pleasant enrichment for children. *It's supporting the development of a nervous system that is more resilient to stress, more capable of sustained attention, and better equipped to regulate emotion.*

## The Silence That Isn't Silent

I want to address something that comes up whenever people start paying attention to natural soundscapes: the mistaken belief that natural environments are quiet.

*They're not.* Stand in a healthy forest at midday in spring and the sound level is surprisingly high—birds calling from multiple directions, insects buzzing in the undergrowth, wind moving through canopy layers at different heights, the creak of branches, and the rustle of small animals in the leaf litter. These environments are acoustically rich. What they lack is a different type of sound—the *specific category of mechanical, artificial, unpredictable sound* that human threat-detection systems flag as potentially dangerous.

Researchers use the term *soundscape* to capture this distinction. A soundscape is the full acoustic environment of a place—everything you can hear, understood as a system rather than a collection of individual sounds; it's like a sound soup. The discipline of soundscape ecology, pioneered by Bernie Krause, has produced a framework for understanding how healthy natural soundscapes are organized: *geophony* (non-biological natural sounds like wind and water), *biophony* (sounds from living organisms), and *anthrophony* (sounds from human activity).

The key insight from this framework is that *healthy natural soundscapes have specific structural properties*—patterns of geophony and biophony that evolved together over millions of years and that human nervous systems evolved alongside. When those patterns are intact, the nervous system reads the environment as healthy and safe. When they're disrupted by anthrophony, *the system's threat-detection mechanisms activate.*

Bernie Krause has spent decades recording natural soundscapes around the world and documenting how they've changed as human activity has increased. In areas of habitat degradation, the loss of biophony—the loss of birdsong, insect chorus, frog calls—is acoustically measurable and ecologically significant. It's also psychologically significant. The increasingly impoverished soundscapes of degraded natural environments *may contribute to the reduced well-being benefits* that some researchers have found in low-quality urban green spaces compared to richer natural settings.

*Quality* of a natural soundscape matters, not just the *quantity* of green space. A park with rich birdsong and running water is likely to be more restorative than a park with the same square footage of grass but little wildlife sound. When you're choosing where to spend outdoor time, *pay attention to what you can hear.*

## Practical Listening: Making Sound Work for You

All of this research converges on something practical: the acoustic environment you inhabit matters for your mental and physical health. And unlike many factors in our environment, it's one *you have more control over than you might think.* When we're thinking of health whether physical or mental we need to consider the level and degree of control we have over various aspects of our lives, including sound.

**The most important step** is the obvious one: *get outside where natural sound is present.* Even urban parks with a good tree canopy tend to have birdsong in the early morning. Water features in city parks provide the acoustic benefits of moving water. Weekends in genuinely natural settings—forests, coasts, and the countryside—provide the fullest version of what natural soundscapes offer. *These experiences accumulate.* You are, over time, recalibrating your nervous system's baseline through regular exposure to sounds that your physiology is built for. Right now, as I sit in a room in my home, I can see trees that are beginning to grow new leaves and a pair of birds that are tending their new ones in a nest in the roof of our building. Yes, the birds are chirping to one another and it's a beautiful spring day with a blue sky and a slight breeze. Everything is coming together as it should in the natural soundscape.

**The second step** is to actually listen. Most of us walk through natural environments with earbuds in, processing podcasts or music while the natural soundscape passes by unheard. I understand the appeal—our relationship with constant audio input has become deeply habitual. But earbuds in a forest or a park means *you're missing exactly the input your nervous system is there to receive.* Can you imagine paying for something so that you will actually miss the most important part of it? It sounds like a waste of your money to me.

*Try leaving the earbuds out for part of your outdoor time.* Not all of it, if that feels too disruptive to your routine. But *even ten minutes* of genuinely attending to the sounds around you—identifying what you hear, noticing how many distinct sound sources you can pick out, paying attention to the layers of sound at different distances—produces measurably different outcomes than the same ten minutes spent listening to something from your phone. The active engagement with natural sound is part of what makes it restorative. In exercise programs, they are now beginning to talk about "snacks," meaning small bits of exercise for a few minutes. I think we might also use the term for "**environmental snacks**." By that I mean just a few minutes in the natural environment, so that you can have the benefit of all of it in *perhaps five or ten minutes' time.*

**The third step** involves your indoor environment, particularly sleep. If you live in a noisy area, the research on pink noise and sleep quality is relevant and actionable. High-quality recordings of natural soundscapes—rain, streams, ocean, and forest—can be used as sleep audio with genuine physiological benefit. This isn't the same as being in nature, but it's *not merely a placebo either*. The frequency properties of natural sound recordings are preserved even when the recordings are played back through speakers, and the brain responds to them accordingly. Many people find that switching from fan-based white noise to natural soundscape recordings improves their sleep quality noticeably within a few days.

**The fourth step** is awareness of your noise environment overall. You probably can't eliminate traffic noise from your life entirely, but you can make choices at the margins—a quieter route on your lunchtime walk, a park bench away from the road, earbuds use specifically during unavoidably noisy commutes as a protective measure rather than habit. Small choices about acoustic environment, made consistently, add up to meaningful differences in the day-to-day load on your nervous system.

As I sit here writing now, a starling is calling to its chicks, which are answering back with a slightly different sound. They are letting the parent know they are there and waiting to be fed. The parent sits patiently in the tree, waiting for the other part of the pair to return with food so this one can go out hunting to feed the chicks too.

When it goes quiet, I know that the local hawk has arrived for his twice-a-day visit.

**And the fifth step**, perhaps *the most underrated:* learn the birds in your area. You don't have to become a birder. You don't need binoculars or field guides or any particular expertise. But knowing the names of a handful of the birds whose songs you hear regularly transforms your relationship with natural sound. It shifts the experience *from passive ambient noise to active recognition*. There are *apps that will identify a bird by its song in real time*—Merlin, from the Cornell Lab of Ornithology, **is free** and remarkably accurate. When you hear a sound and your brain connects it to something specific and known, the sense of relationship with the environment deepens. That relationship, research increasingly shows, *is itself therapeutic.* Undoubtedly, it's therapy without the expense.

## The Quiet Case for Awe

There's one final dimension of natural sound that doesn't fit neatly into the physiological categories we've been discussing, but that deserves a place in this chapter anyway.

Some natural soundscapes don't just calm you. *They move you.*

The sound of a thunderstorm from inside a cabin. The ocean in heavy surf. A chorus of frogs after summer rain. A forest at night alive with insect sound. These acoustic experiences produce something beyond relaxation—something that researchers who *study the emotion of awe* describe as a sense of vastness, of being small in relationship to something much larger, of ordinary categories dissolving briefly.

Looking up at the sky on one of those starry nights in Rhode Island, I remember being surprised that there were so many stars I had never seen before. Of course, part of the problem was that I live near a major city that blocks out any view of the night sky that includes all of the stars visible in the Rhode Island area. I was awestruck.

Awe is a distinct emotional state that has been the subject of serious scientific study for about two decades, largely due to the work of psychologist Dacher Keltner at UC Berkeley. Awe, Keltner's research has found, produces specific physiological effects: *reduced inflammation markers, increased vagal tone (a measure of parasympathetic nervous system health), reduced self-focused thinking, and increased prosocial behavior.* Children also benefit from a sense of awe in terms of learning. People who experience awe regularly show greater life satisfaction and greater resilience to stress than those who rarely experience it.

Natural soundscapes—particularly the large-scale, immersive acoustic experiences that only come from being inside a genuinely wild environment—are among the *most reliable triggers of awe that exist.* This may be one reason why people who spend time in truly natural settings often describe feeling changed by the experience in ways that go beyond what better mood and lower cortisol can fully account for. Something has shifted in their sense of themselves and their relationship to the world.

That shift is real. It's measurable. And it may be available to you more often than you realize if you're willing to put down the earbuds, step into the sound, and actually listen to what's there.

## What's Coming Next

In the first six chapters of this book, we've examined the outdoor environment through five senses: *what you breathe, what you smell, what you see (light and water), how you move, and what you hear*. In each case, the research tells the same story—your brain and body were built for a natural environment, and giving ourselves access to that environment, even in small doses, produces measurable changes in the systems that govern mood, stress, cognition, and health.

In Chapter 7, we're going to tackle something different. We're going to look at the social dimension of time in nature more deeply—specifically at loneliness, isolation, and what the research says about how natural environments change the way we connect with other people. Because it turns out that getting outside doesn't just change your internal state. *It changes how you show up in relationships, how open you feel toward strangers, and how connected you feel to something beyond yourself.*

And for a world that is *dealing with a loneliness epidemic* that mental health professionals are increasingly describing as a *public health crisis*, that matters more than most of us realize.

## CHAPTER 6 REFERENCES

Alkaya Karagoz M, Altundogan S. The effect of music and white noise on patients' anxiety and pain during surgery for impacted mandibular third molars: a single-blind randomized controlled trial. Eur J Med Res. 2025 Jun 23;30(1):506. doi: 10.1186/s40001-025-02767-1. PMID: 40551282; PMCID: PMC12183815.

Alvarsson, J. J., Wiens, S., & Nilsson, M. E. (2010). Stress recovery during exposure to nature sound and environmental noise. International Journal of Environmental Research and Public Health, 7(3), 1036–1046. https://doi.org/10.3390/ijerph7031036

eClinicalMedicine. The epidemic of loneliness. EClinicalMedicine. 2023 Dec 15;66:102395. doi: 10.1016/j.eclinm.2023.102395. PMID: 38192594; PMCID: PMC10772224.

Evans, G. W., & Lepore, S. J. (1993). Nonauditory effects of noise on children: A critical review. Children's Environments, 10(1), 31–51. https://www.jstor.org/stable/41514773

Ferrario, M., Piccolo, E., Lanzini, M., De Mita, A. C., & Giannattasio, C. (2021). Physiological effects of natural sound on surgical recovery. Pain Medicine, 22(11), 2517–2526. https://doi.org/10.1093/pm/pnab142

Gidlow, C. J., Jones, M. V., Hurst, G., Masterson, D., Clark-Carter, D., Tarvainen, M. P., Smith, G., & Nieuwenhuijsen, M. (2016). Where to find nature's lead? A systematic review and meta-analysis of green exercise and mental health outcomes. British Journal of Sports Medicine, 50(18), 1176–1183. https://doi.org/10.1136/bjsports-2015-095687

Gopal KV, Mills LE, Phillips BS, Nandy R. Risk Assessment of Recreational Noise-Induced Hearing Loss from Exposure through a Personal Audio System-iPod Touch. J Am Acad Audiol. 2019 Jul/Aug;30(7):619-633. doi: 10.3766/jaaa.17140. Epub 2018 Nov 1. PMID: 30395532.

Hammoud, R., Tognin, S., Burgess, L., Bergou, N., Smythe, M., Gibbons, J., Davidson, N., Afifi, A., Bakolis, I., & Bhome, R. (2022). Smartphone-based ecological momentary assessment reveals mental health benefits of birdlife. Scientific Reports, 12, 17589. https://doi .org/10.1038/s41598-022-20207-6

Keltner, D. (2023). Awe: The new science of everyday wonder and how it can transform your life. Penguin Press. https://dacherkeltner .com/awe-book

Krause, B. (2012). The great animal orchestra: Finding the origins of music in the world's wild places. Little, Brown and Company. https://www.berniemkrause.com/publications

Laszlo, H. E., McRobie, E. S., Stansfeld, S. A., & Hansell, A. L. (2012). Residential road traffic noise and mental health: An urban perspective with new evidence on annoyance. Noise & Health, 14(58), 99–107. https://doi.org/10.4103/1463-1741.95138

Medvedev, O., Shepherd, D., & Hautus, M. J. (2015). The restorative potential of soundscapes: A physiological investigation. Applied Acoustics, 96, 20–26. https://doi.org/10.1016/j.apacoust.2015.03. 004

O'bi A, Yang F. Seeing awe: How children perceive awe-inspiring visual experiences. Child Dev. 2024 Jul-Aug;95(4):1271-1286. doi: 10.1111/cdev.14069. Epub 2024 Jan 31. PMID: 38294048.

Peen, J., Schoevers, R. A., Beekman, A. T., & Dekker, J. (2010). The current status of urban-rural differences in psychiatric disorders. Acta Psychiatrica Scandinavica, 121(2), 84–93. https://doi.org/10.1111/ j.1600-0447.2009.01438.x

Schroeer A, Corona-Strauss FI, Hannemann R, Hackley SA and Strauss DJ (2025) Electromyographic correlates of effortful listening in the vestigial auriculomotor system. Front. Neurosci. 18:1462507. doi: 10.3389/fnins.2024.1462507

Sueur, Jérôme & Krause, Bernie & Farina, Almo. (2021). Acoustic biodiversity. Current biology: CB. 31. R1172-R1173. 10.1016/j.cu b.2021.08.063.

Tao, J., Li, X., Stenfors, C. U. D., Rumble, A., & Nilsson, M. E. (2021). Effects of birdsong on urban residents' restoration. Environmental Research, 195, 110299. https://doi.org/10.1016/j.envres.20 20.110299

Thoma MV, Mewes R, Nater UM. Preliminary evidence: the stress-reducing effect of listening to water sounds depends on somatic complaints: A randomized trial. Medicine (Baltimore). 2018 Feb;97(8):e9851. doi: 10.1097/MD.0000000000009851. PMID: 29465568; PMCID: PMC5842016.

WHO Regional Office for Europe. (2018). Environmental noise guidelines for the European region. World Health Organization. https://www.euro.who.int/en/publications/abstracts/environ mental-noise-guidelines-for-the-european-region-2018

Zhou, X., Rosini, J. M., & Bhatt, D. L. (2023). Long-term traffic noise exposure and risk of depression: A population-based study of two million adults. The Lancet Regional Health – Americas, 18, 100406. https://doi.org/10.1016/j.lana.2022.1004

# Chapter 7: The Loneliness Cure: How Nature Changes the Way We Connect with Other People

## The Epidemic Nobody Wants to Talk About

We are living through *a loneliness crisis*. I know that's hard to believe when we think of how many millions of people there are in the United States and how many opportunities for friendship that must create.

How could we possibly be lonely, especially if we are living in cities that are teeming with millions of people? However, *loneliness is pervasive*, and the presence of millions of people around us doesn't diminish it. It's a plague of a sort that healthcare is currently attempting to tackle. Recall that one of the recent Surgeon Generals of the United States indicated that he and his staff believed that loneliness was creating an incredible crisis in our country. The Surgeon General said it was more than a crisis; **it was an epidemic.**

That's not a dramatic statement. It's the conclusion of public health researchers, government health agencies, and mental health professionals across multiple countries who have been tracking the data for years. In 2023, the United States Surgeon General *issued a formal advisory calling loneliness and social isolation a public health epidemic*, citing research showing that approximately *half of American adults report measurable levels of loneliness* and that the health consequences of that loneliness are severe enough to be *compared, in terms of mortality risk, to smoking fifteen cigarettes a day.* We know that loneliness would be associated with heightened stress and stress depletes the immune system, which would make it much more vulnerable to developing cancer or other illnesses.

*Fifteen cigarettes a day*. We've built entire public health campaigns around the dangers of smoking. We put warning labels on cigarette packages. We taxed tobacco and banned advertising directed at children. And yet a condition that carries comparable mortality risk *has received a fraction of that public attention,* a fraction of that policy response, and *almost no practical guidance* for ordinary people about what to actually do about it.

In the United Kingdom, the problem was deemed serious enough that the government appointed a *Minister for Loneliness* in 2018—a dedicated cabinet position whose entire purpose was addressing social isolation as a national health emergency. Other countries have followed. The research that prompted these responses is unambiguous: **chronic loneliness raises the risk of premature death**, increases the risk of heart disease, stroke, dementia, depression, and anxiety, impairs immune function, disrupts sleep, and accelerates cognitive decline in older adults. How much more evidence do we need to underscore the importance and the seriousness of loneliness as a health issue?

*Loneliness isn't a feeling to be managed. It is a physiological state with consequences as real as any chronic disease.*

So what does any of this have to do with going outside? More than you might expect.

One of the most consistent and robust findings in natural environment research is that it *changes how humans relate*. They reduce defensiveness. They increase trust. They make people more willing to engage with strangers. It creates the conditions in which real human connection—the kind that actually resolves loneliness at a physiological level—is more likely to happen.

On the morning of 9/11, I was working in an office building. At 11:00 AM, all of us decided to leave because a national emergency was taking place. As I left the building to go to a parking garage for my car, a woman came walking down the street and we began to talk to each other as though we had been friends. When we parted, we wished each other a safe trip home that day. I'm sure that happened to many people with many strangers. The attack created a sense of togetherness with strangers.

This chapter is about why loneliness is such a major problem and what you can do about it.

## What Loneliness Actually Does to the Body

Before we explore the solution, it helps to understand the problem clearly. Loneliness is more than just feeling sad because you don't have enough friends. *It's a biological state* with a specific physiological profile, and understanding that profile helps explain why the things that reduce it—including time in nature—work the way they do.

The neuroscientist John Cacioppo spent decades studying loneliness and its biological effects, and his findings are some of the most important in modern psychology. Cacioppo found that loneliness activates a specific set of biological responses that mirror, in many ways, the body's response to physical threat. *Lonely people show elevated cortisol.* They show *increased inflammatory markers*. They show heightened activity in the amygdala—*the brain's alarm center*—and *increased sensitivity to social threat cues*. Their brains are, in the most literal sense, on high alert. Anyone maintaining that high level of alert is taxing their body's ability to remain healthy and predisposing it to illness.

This makes evolutionary sense. For a social species like us, being separated from the group was genuinely dangerous. A human being alone, separated from the tribe, was vulnerable to predators, starvation, and injury in ways that a person embedded in a social group wasn't. The pain of loneliness—the real, physical discomfort of it—evolved as a *signal to motivate reconnection*, the same way hunger motivates eating and thirst motivates drinking.

But here's the **cruel paradox** that Cacioppo identified: *loneliness changes the brain in ways that make reconnection harder.* Lonely people become *hypervigilant for social threats*. They expect rejection. They interpret ambiguous social signals negatively. They become more likely to perceive neutral interactions as hostile and to withdraw from situations that might offer connection. The biological state of loneliness, if sustained long enough, *actively undermines the behaviors that would resolve it.*

This is why telling a lonely person to just go out and socialize more is *roughly as useful as telling a depressed person to cheer up.* The condition itself *changes the internal environment* in ways that make the obvious remedy feel impossible. In effect, the individual is trying now to fight a biological imperative to remain isolated. What can we do about that?

What's needed is *something that reduces the threat-detection hyperactivation first*—something that brings the nervous system down from high alert before social engagement is attempted. And this is exactly where natural environments enter the picture.

## How Nature Lowers Your Social Defenses

Natural environments have a *measurable and consistent effect on the vigilance systems that loneliness amplifies.* We've talked throughout this book about how nature activates the parasympathetic nervous system, reduces cortisol, and calms amygdala activity. **All of those effects apply here**, and they matter specifically for social connection because a calm nervous system is more open and trusting.

When your stress response is activated—when you're in fight-or-flight mode, when your cortisol is elevated, when your amygdala is scanning for threats—your social processing *shifts toward self-protection. You read other people's faces for signs of danger.* You interpret ambiguity as hostility. You become more likely to see out-group members as threatening and less likely to feel generosity toward strangers. This is adaptive when the threat is real. It's profoundly counterproductive when the threat is loneliness itself.

*Time in natural environments reverses this pattern*. A 2014 study published in the journal Environment and Behavior found that people who spent time walking in natural settings showed significantly greater prosocial behavior—willingness to help strangers, generosity in resource-sharing tasks, and positive attributions about other people's intentions—than people who spent equivalent time in urban settings. The nature walkers were, in measurable terms, more open to other people. And this isn't the only study that provided hopeful information.

A 2019 study from the University of Rochester extended this finding by examining what they called *nature connectedness*—the sense of feeling part of the natural world—and its relationship to prosocial values and generosity. Participants who were primed to feel connected to nature showed increased empathy, greater concern for others' well-being, and greater willingness to act in ways that benefited other people at a cost to themselves. The mechanism appeared to involve a *shift from self-focused processing to other-focused* processing that the experience of natural environments reliably triggers. How does this happen?

Think about what this means practically. Natural environments don't just make you feel better. They make you a better social actor—more open, more generous, more willing to connect. And they do this by changing the same physiological systems that loneliness dysregulates. In a very real sense, time in nature prepares the nervous system for genuine human connection in ways that our current indoor, screen-mediated, artificial-environment lives don't.

## Soft Fascination and the Open Mind

There's a specific *psychological mechanism at work* here that's worth naming: what *attention restoration* theorists Rachel and Stephen Kaplan called *soft fascination*.

We discussed attention restoration theory briefly in Chapter 1. The Kaplans proposed that natural environments restore depleted attentional capacity through a specific quality they called *soft fascination*—the kind of gentle, effortless attention that a natural setting demands. Watching clouds move, following the path of a stream, and noticing birds. These things hold your attention without requiring directed, effortful focus. They occupy the mind gently, without depleting it.

*Directed attention*—the kind you use *when you're working*, solving problems, driving in traffic, or navigating a complex social environment—is an effortful, limited resource. It depletes our mental energy with use and requires genuine rest to restore. When your directed attention is depleted, your capacity for emotional regulation, impulse control, patience, and thoughtful social engagement depletes along with it. *You become snappier, more reactive, less tolerant, and less able to be genuinely present with other people.*

*Soft fascination* restores directed attention without effort. You're not trying to rest. You're simply in an environment that allows restoration to happen. And as that restoration occurs, something interesting happens to your relationship with other people: *you become more present with them.*

The research on attention restoration and interpersonal quality is suggestive and compelling. Studies have found that people who spend time in natural settings before social interactions report those interactions as feeling more meaningful, more satisfying, and more genuinely connecting than interactions that follow time in urban or indoor environments. The nature time doesn't just make you calmer.

*It makes you a better listener, a more patient conversation partner, and a more present human being.* A major part of being present in any relationship is that you are a good listener and attentive to what other people are saying or implying.

For anyone who has experienced the feeling of being truly listened to—really heard by someone who was fully there with you—and compared it to the experience of talking to someone who is clearly somewhere else in their head, the significance of such interactions is obvious. Presence is the core ingredient of genuine human connection. And nature restores it.

## Shared Nature and the Bond It Creates

There's something special about experiencing a natural environment with another person who seems to create connection in ways that other shared experiences don't replicate as reliably. Ask anyone who has ever hiked with a close friend, sat with a family member watching the sun set, or walked through a forest with someone they love. The shared experience of nature has a quality of intimacy that is challenging to manufacture in other settings.

Research supports this intuition. A 2020 study published in the Journal of Environmental Psychology found that pairs of people who completed a walk in a natural setting reported greater feelings of closeness and connection afterward than pairs who completed the same walk in an urban setting—even though the conversations during the walks were similar in length and content. *The environment influenced the relational experience* beyond what the conversation itself produced.

One factor appears to be what researchers call **shared awe**. When two people are simultaneously exposed to something that produces awe—a vast landscape, a dramatic natural phenomenon, or the sheer biological richness of a healthy forest—the experience of that awe is itself bonding. Dacher Keltner's research on awe, which we touched on in Chapter 6, includes findings that awe experienced in the presence of others increases feelings of affiliation and social connection more strongly than awe experienced alone.

Another factor is the way that natural settings *reduce social performance pressure*. Like it or not, if you give it some thought, every single human interaction is a performance of one type or another. Indoor social environments—parties, restaurants, offices—require a degree of social management. *You're performing in the sociological sense*. You're *monitoring* how you come across, *managing impressions*, and *navigating the implicit rules* of the social setting.

Natural environments reduce this performance pressure. *There is less of a social script to follow*. Is there even a social script you have to follow when you're out in nature? The environment itself provides shared focus that doesn't require either person to entertain the other. You can be together while both attending to the same beautiful or interesting third thing, and that parallel attention to a shared world creates a different kind of companionship than face-to-face conversation requires.

For people who find social interaction exhausting—introverts, people with social anxiety, people who are socially out of practice after years of isolation—this reduction in performance pressure can be the difference between connection that actually happens and connection that remains perpetually deferred.

## The Stranger Problem: Why We Stop Talking to Each Other

One of the most striking features of modern urban life is how thoroughly *we have stopped talking to strangers.* On public transit, in elevators, in waiting rooms and coffee shops—the default is silence, phones out, eyes down, and social contact systematically avoided. This is a relatively recent norm. It has developed alongside smartphones, earbuds, and the general overabundance of public space that limits us. But we also have to consider the glut of mainstream media that *emphasizes the dangers in our culture* and this has a tremendous effect on us. And the mental health consequences of it are more significant than most people realize.

Research by Nicholas Epley at the University of Chicago has documented what he calls *the mistaken belief that strangers don't want to be spoken to.* In study after study, Epley found that people *systematically underestimate how much strangers enjoy being engaged in conversation*. People predict that talking to a stranger on a train will be awkward and unrewarding. The actual experience, when researchers prompt people to try it, is almost universally more positive than predicted. People report feeling better, more connected, and more positive about their day after conversations with strangers—even brief ones—than after riding in silence.

The problem is that the social environment of modern urban life makes initiating those conversations feel risky in a way that the social environment of natural settings doesn't.

Natural environments, research consistently shows, increase what sociologists call *incidental social contact*—brief, pleasant interactions with people you encounter in shared space. Neighbors talking across the fence. Dog owners chatting while their dogs interact. People on a trail offering each other a good morning. Park-goers making eye contact and smiling at something a child is doing. These interactions are small. They don't require vulnerability or commitment. But they accumulate into something that matters: *the sense that the social world is basically friendly*, that other people are approachable, that you are not isolated even when you're technically alone. These days, we often hear on social media that our culture is sick and that evil is pandemic. This is counter to what we would like to believe about the world we live in. We don't live in a sick world. We live in a world that is constantly pushing toward alienation.

A landmark study by William Sullivan and colleagues at the University of Illinois examined residents of a large public housing project. Buildings with more green space and trees surrounding them showed significantly higher rates of social contact among neighbors, stronger social ties, and greater community cohesion than otherwise comparable buildings with less green space. The green spaces were creating the conditions for the incidental contacts that build community. They were providing a reason to be outside and a shared, pleasant environment that made interaction feel natural rather than forced. When you think about this research, reconsider what major cities have traditionally built in terms of low-cost housing for thousands of families. What they have actually created was a situation where loneliness and suspicion of strangers or even neighbors were developing by the very architecture they were planning.

One major example would be the work of *Robert Moses* when he constructed the Cross-Bronx Expressway in New York City and *destroyed communities*, replacing them with high-rise projects. What resulted wasn't only a loss of friendships and integrated community relationships as the highway tore through the middle of the community, but also an increase in crime as residents felt disconnected from their living spaces and their neighbors. People who had once lived next to their neighbors in familiar one-and two-family houses now found they were separated from them by a highway with six lanes.

This finding has been replicated across different populations and settings. Green spaces in urban environments don't just improve individual mental health. *They build the social fabric of communities.* They create the *conditions under which neighbors become neighbors* rather than strangers who happen to live near each other.

## Nature and the Loneliest Among Us

While outdoor environments benefit essentially everyone's social well-being, the effects are largest and most clinically meaningful for the people who are most severely isolated. *Several specific populations deserve mention.*

**Older adults** face the highest rates of severe, chronic loneliness in most developed countries. They are often dealing with the cumulative losses of aging—the death of spouses, the departure of children, retirement from work communities, reduced mobility—at exactly the time when their physical and cognitive health most requires social support. The research on nature-based programs for older adults is both well-established and underutilized.

A 2020 systematic review published in the journal Health and Place analyzed seventeen studies of nature-based interventions for older adults and found consistent improvements in loneliness, social connection, sense of purpose, and mental well-being. Community gardening programs, walking groups in parks, and horticulture therapy programs all produced significant effects. Crucially, these programs worked not only by getting older adults into natural settings but also by *creating structured social opportunities within those settings*—giving people a shared purpose and a shared environment that made connection feel natural rather than forced.

**People recovering from addiction** represent another population for whom nature-based social programming has shown particular promise. Recovery requires rebuilding a social world from scratch—*replacing the social networks built around substance use with new connections and new communities.* Natural settings have been used effectively in recovery programs as venues for group activities that create sober social bonds, and the evidence suggests that the calming, trust-enhancing effects of natural environments may be specifically helpful for people whose social trust has been damaged by the experiences that accompany addiction. We've seen some of these rehabilitation programs on TV. One in particular deals with pit bull rehabilitation. These dogs were seen as pariahs but in rehabilitating them, the individuals involved found a new purpose and a means toward greater social connection.

**Young adults**—who, counterintuitively, now report higher rates of loneliness than older age groups in many surveys—face a particular challenge in the current social environment. Social media creates the appearance of connection without many of its physiological benefits. Seeing other people's lives on a screen *doesn't produce the co-regulation of nervous systems that genuine in-person contact provides*. Research by Jean Twenge and others has documented a generation spending more time online and on screens, less time in face-to-face social contact, and showing markedly higher rates of anxiety, depression, and loneliness than previous generations at comparable ages. You have to wonder what the newfound "friendships" with avatars on computers will bring to the younger generation.

For young adults, the case for outdoor social activity is **particularly compelling.** The research suggests that nature-based social experiences—hiking groups, outdoor sports, community gardens, and trail volunteering—provide exactly the combination that this population needs: genuine in-person contact, shared physical experience, reduced performance pressure, and the physiological grounding that screen time actively undermines.

## The Sense of Belonging to Something Larger

There's a dimension of the nature-loneliness relationship that goes beyond individual human connections, and that the most comprehensive researchers in this field have started to take seriously: the relationship between nature connectedness and the sense of belonging to something larger than oneself.

Loneliness, at its deepest level, isn't simply about the absence of other people. *It's about a sense of disconnection*—from other people, yes, but also from meaning, from purpose, from the feeling that one's existence is part of something that matters. *Purpose is one thing that gives life meaning* and has been found to be central to keeping people healthy. This disconnection is a deeper form of existential isolation that can persist even in people who have adequate social contact, and it can be just as damaging as the social variety.

Time in natural environments addresses this form of loneliness through what researchers call *nature connectedness*—a sense of kinship with the living world, of being embedded in biological systems that extend far beyond the human. This isn't a mystical or religious claim. It is a psychological one, and it is measurable.

Miles Richardson and his colleagues at the University of Derby have developed a validated measure of nature connectedness and have spent years studying its relationship to well-being. Their research consistently finds that people who score higher on nature connectedness—who feel a sense of relationship with the natural world, who notice and appreciate natural things, who feel that they are part of nature rather than separate from it—show *higher levels of psychological well-being, greater life satisfaction, lower anxiety, and lower depression.* The relationship is robust and holds across different populations and different measures.

Importantly, nature connectedness is not the same as time spent outdoors. It's a qualitative shift in how a person relates to the natural world—*a shift from seeing nature as scenery to experiencing it as community.* And that shift appears to be something that *can be cultivated deliberately*, through the kinds of attentive, engaged outdoor experiences this book is describing.

When you start to notice the birds, learn their names, and recognize the trees and observe the insects—when the natural world becomes populated with particulars that you know and recognize—something changes in your relationship to it. You are no longer a visitor in a landscape. You are a resident. And that sense of being known by and knowing a place, of belonging somewhere on this earth, is an antidote to existential loneliness that no amount of social media engagement can replicate. I recall a squirrel that was running around the grounds of our large complex. One thing that distinguished it from others was that *it had no tail.* I called it "Bunny." When I saw Bunny, I would call and stand with a peanut in my hand. Gradually, the squirrel would approach me, run to my side, settle at my feet, and take the nut. I was incredibly connected to that wild animal.

## Biophilia and the Longing We Don't Have a Name For

In Chapter 1, we introduced the concept of biophilia—E.O. Wilson's term for the innate human tendency to affiliate with other living systems. Here, I want to revisit that concept from a social angle, because *biophilia isn't just about individual well-being.* It's about where humans find their deepest sense of membership.

For most of human history, the community that people belonged to wasn't separate from the natural world. The tribe lived in a particular place, with particular animals and plants, particular seasons and weather patterns and ecological rhythms. Everything was pretty much predictable. The human social community and the biological community were intertwined in ways that are almost impossible for modern people to fully imagine.

We saw what happened in the United States, in Oklahoma, when people dismissed the Native Americans' understanding of the land, ripped it up, and replaced it with crops that, after a few years, failed, leaving *what we now know as "The Dust Bowl."* The loss of that embeddedness—the disembedding of human social life from the natural world that industrialization and urbanization produced—is one of the least-discussed and perhaps most significant losses of the modern era. Climate change could well be our century's version of the Dust Bowl.

Wilson argued that this disembedding produces a specific kind of psychological suffering: a longing for the natural world that modern people experience without being able to name it. The restlessness. The sense that something is missing. The way vacations in natural settings feel disproportionately restorative, as though you've been given back something you didn't know had been taken. There is a mental hunger and thirst for these settings and the relationships that come from them. That feeling isn't nostalgia for childhood or romanticism about the past. It is a genuine *response to deprivation* of something the human organism needs.

Understanding loneliness through this lens changes what solutions look like. It's not just about adding more social engagements to your calendar. It's about reconnecting with the web of living things that your nervous system was built to inhabit—and allowing the communities you find there, human and otherwise, to anchor you in the world *in the way that you were designed to be anchored.*

When I was a little girl, we had the misfortune of living in a cold-water flat on the second floor. In front of the row house, there was only dirt—not even a blade of grass—and behind us, the same thing. My mother brought into our home two types of flowering plants that could easily live in our little apartment: a crown of thorns and a wax begonia. Both thrived and that was our connection with nature. Later we would have the good fortune to rent a home where my mother and sisters planted flowers in front of the house and rose bushes in the yard. People waiting for the bus would sometimes take one of our flowers. It was a small price to pay for the abundance of flowers that grew there. We were connected with those flowers and every single member of my extended family has a garden.

## Making It Real: Practical Paths to Connection Through Nature

All of the above have practical implications, and I want to end this chapter with specific, actionable suggestions—because understanding why nature helps with loneliness isn't enough. *You need to know what to actually do.*

**The first,** and most important, thing is to find a regular outdoor spot and make it yours. Research on place attachment—the psychological bond between a person and a specific location—finds that having a place you return to regularly, where you recognize the seasonal changes and the regular wildlife and the rhythms of the environment, produces a sense of rootedness and belonging that is *directly antithetical to loneliness.* This doesn't have to be a dramatic landscape. It can be a neighborhood park, a particular trail, a community garden plot, a stretch of waterfront. *What matters is regularity and attention.*

**The second thing** is to find outdoor activities that *have a social structure built in*. Joining a walking group, a hiking club, a birdwatching society, a community garden, a photography group, an outdoor yoga class, or a trail maintenance volunteer program places you in the company of other people in a natural setting, with a shared purpose, and without the performance pressure of purely social events. *The shared activity does much of the relational work*. You don't have to be witty or interesting. You just have to show up and participate.

**The third thing** is to practice what's called *slow outdoor attention*—the deliberate act of noticing the specific, particular things in your outdoor environment, rather than passing through it. What birds are in that tree? What are those small plants growing in the cracks of the path? I check for the appearance of really tiny wildflowers, violets and wild strawberries in the vast lawns in our complex. I take photos with my cell and post the flower photos online on social media for everyone to share. Also, what does the air smell like today compared to last week? This practice, beyond its individual benefits, gives you something to share with other people. Noticing things together is one of the most natural forms of human bonding. It's what children do spontaneously and *what adults have largely forgotten*. It doesn't require conversation skills. It just requires paying attention out loud.

**The fourth thing** is to *say "good* morning." This sounds embarrassingly simple. It is also genuinely powerful. Research by Nicholas Epley and others shows that brief, friendly interactions with strangers—which are far more common in outdoor natural settings than in most indoor environments—accumulate into a meaningful sense of social connection over time. The person you nod at on the trail. The neighbor you stop for thirty seconds to admire the garden with. The dog owner you chat with while your dogs sniff each other is friendly. Even the young man attempting to select fruit in an outdoor market. *These interactions are not trivial.* They are the social connective tissue that makes a life feel embedded rather than isolated.

**The fifth thing** is to bring someone with you. Not always—solo time in nature has its own value, and there are experiences that require solitude. But the research on shared nature experiences is unambiguous: doing this with another person, even occasionally, produces relational benefits that solo time doesn't. If you're lonely, the temptation is to withdraw. Nature gives you an excuse to reach out—not for a deep, vulnerable conversation, but for a walk. A walk is manageable. A walk with someone else is both manageable and connecting.

*Loneliness is a signal.* It tells you that something the human organism needs is missing. The research we've explored in this chapter suggests that natural environments offer a remarkably direct response to that signal—by calming the nervous system, reducing social defensiveness, creating conditions for incidental connection, and restoring the deeper sense of belonging to a world that extends beyond any individual human life.

You weren't designed to be isolated. You were designed to belong to a community of people and to a community of living things that is larger than any room you have ever been in.

Get outside. Find your place. Let yourself belong to it.

## What's Coming Next

We've now covered seven chapters exploring how the outdoor environment shapes your mental and physical health through air, scent, water, light, movement, sound, and social connection. In Chapter 8, we'll turn our attention to a question that comes up inevitably whenever this subject is discussed: *What about people who can't easily get outside?*

*Physical disability, chronic illness, urban density, weather, safety concerns, demanding schedules*—these are real barriers, and dismissing them isn't useful. Chapter 8 will look honestly at those barriers and at the research on what works when full outdoor access isn't possible—from window views and houseplants to green urban design and virtual nature—while making the case that access to nature isn't a luxury but a health equity issue that deserves serious attention.

The benefits described in this book *shouldn't be available only to those who are young, healthy, mobile, and affluent.* They should be available to everyone. And increasingly, thoughtful people are working to make that happen.

## CHAPTER 7 REFERENCES

Alexander R, Nugent C, Nugent K. The Dust Bowl in the US: An Analysis Based on Current Environmental and Clinical Studies. Am J Med Sci. 2018 Aug;356(2):90-96. doi: 10.1016/j.amjms.2018.03.015. Epub 2018 Mar 26. PMID: 30219167.

Cacioppo, J. T., & Patrick, W. (2008). Loneliness: Human nature and the need for social connection. W.W. Norton & Company. https://www.amazon.com/Loneliness-Human-Nature-Need-Connection/dp/0393335283

Epley, N., & Schroeder, J. (2014). Mistakenly seeking solitude. Journal of Experimental Psychology: General, 143(5), 1980–1999. https://doi.org/10.1037/a0037323

Holt-Lunstad, J., Smith, T. B., Baker, M., Harris, T., & Stephenson, D. (2015). Loneliness and social isolation as risk factors for mortality: A meta-analytic review. Perspectives on Psychological Science, 10(2), 227–237. https://doi.org/10.1177/1745691614568352

Kaplan, R., & Kaplan, S. (1989). The experience of nature: A psychological perspective. Cambridge University Press. https://doi.org/10.1017/CBO9780511621994

Keltner, D., & Haidt, J. (2003). Approaching awe, a moral, spiritual, and aesthetic emotion. Cognition and Emotion, 17(2), 297–314. https://doi.org/10.1080/02699930302297

Marselle, M. R., Martens, D., Dallimer, M., & Irvine, K. N. (2020). Review of the mental health and well-being benefits of biodiversity. In M. R. Marselle, J. Stadler, H. Korn, K. N. Irvine, & A. Bonn (Eds.), Biodiversity and health in the face of climate change. Springer, Cham. https://doi.org/10.1007/978-3-030-02318-8_10

Office of the Surgeon General (OSG). Our Epidemic of Loneliness and Isolation: The U.S. Surgeon General's Advisory on the Healing Effects of Social Connection and Community [Internet]. Washington (DC): US Department of Health and Human Services; 2023–. PMID: 37792968.

Richardson, M., Cormack, A., McRobert, L., & Underhill, R. (2016). 30 days wild: Development and evaluation of a large-scale nature engagement campaign to improve well-being. PLOS ONE, 11(2), e0149777. https://doi.org/10.1371/journal.pone.0149777

Soga, M., Gaston, K. J., & Yamaura, Y. (2017). Gardening is beneficial for health: A meta-analysis. Preventive Medicine Reports, 5, 92–99. https://doi.org/10.1016/j.pmedr.2016.11.007

Sullivan, W. C., Kuo, F. E., & DePooter, S. F. (2004). The fruit of urban nature: Vital neighborhood spaces. Environment and Behavior, 36(5), 678–700. https://doi.org/10.1177/0193841X04264945

Twenge, J. M. (2017). iGen: Why today's super-connected kids are growing up less rebellious, more tolerant, less happy—and completely unprepared for adulthood. Atria Books. https://www.simonandschuster.com/books/iGen/Jean-M-Twenge/9781501152016

U.S. Department of Health and Human Services. (2023). Our epidemic of loneliness and isolation: The U.S. Surgeon General's advisory on the healing effects of social connection and community. Office of the Surgeon General. https://www.hhs.gov/sites/default/files/surgeon-general-social-connection-advisory.pdf

Wilson, E. O. (1984). Biophilia. Harvard University Press. https://www.hup.harvard.edu/catalog.php?isbn=9780674074422

Zhang, J. W., Howell, R. T., & Iyer, R. (2014). Engagement with natural beauty moderates the positive relation between connectedness with nature and psychological well-being. Journal of Environmental Psychology, 38, 55–63. https://doi.org/10.1016/j.jenvp.2013.12.013

Zilioli S, Slatcher RB, Chi P, Li X, Zhao J, Zhao G. The impact of daily and trait loneliness on diurnal cortisol and sleep among children affected by parental HIV/AIDS. Psychoneuroendocrinology. 2017 Jan;75:64-71. doi: 10.1016/j.psyneuen.2016.10.012. Epub 2016 Oct 25. PMID: 27810705; PMCID: PMC5256636.

# Chapter 8: What If You Can't Get Out? Nature's Benefits When the Door Won't Open

## The Question I Get Asked More Than Any Other

During every talk I give about the mental health benefits of being outdoors, someone raises their hand before I finish speaking. They always ask some version of the same question.

"What about people who can't go outside? What about the person in a wheelchair? The woman with fibromyalgia can barely get off the couch. The man lives in a high-rise apartment in a neighborhood where walking alone at night feels genuinely dangerous. The single mom working two jobs who hasn't had an hour to herself in three months?"

It's a fair question. It's more than fair. It's the most important question anyone can ask in this conversation. Because if everything in this book only applies to people who are healthy, mobile, wealthy, and living near a park, then I haven't written a book about mental health. I've written a book about privilege and that's not my intention. I know what it's like to live without privilege; when we were quite poor, we lived in a slumlord's apartment in rowhouses without heat or hot water. I, as a five-year-old, had to collect darkened coal cinders for my mother to use to make hot water for bathing. Privilege didn't exist in our neighborhood.

So let's talk honestly about barriers. Then let's talk about what the research shows for the millions of people who face them. Because it turns out the story is *more hopeful than you might expect.*

## The Barriers Are Real

First, a word about honesty. *I won't say that outdoor access barriers aren't real* or that they can be easily solved with the right attitude. That kind of advice isn't useful. *It is, in fact, insulting.*

The barriers are real. Let me name them plainly.

*Physical disability* is among the most common. According to a 2025 report published in the journal Frontiers in Public Health, approximately *1.3 billion people worldwide*—about 16 percent of the global population—live with some form of disability. Many of those disabilities directly limit the kind of outdoor activity this book has been describing. A person with severe rheumatoid arthritis, Parkinson's disease, multiple sclerosis, a recent stroke, or a serious spinal injury may face genuine physical barriers to spending time outdoors—barriers that no amount of motivation or willpower will remove.

*Chronic illness* adds another layer. Conditions like lupus, fibromyalgia, severe asthma, heart failure, and chronic fatigue syndrome don't just make outdoor activity difficult. We know that lupus, in particular, can have serious side effects, such as stroke, with repeated exposure to sunshine. I know that chronic fatigue syndrome is a scientific fact. I can tell you that I have worked with physicians who believed it was a way of getting disability payments. These were physicians who made the decisions. It was incredibly cruel and dishonest. These disorders can make it genuinely dangerous to be outdoors. Heat, cold, pollen, uneven terrain, and even the physical exertion of walking to a park can carry real health risks for people living with these conditions.

Then there are the social and environmental barriers. Urban density means that millions of Americans live in neighborhoods without parks, trees, or accessible green space. Bad weather—whether that means January in Minnesota or August in Phoenix—can make outdoor time genuinely unpleasant or hazardous for months at a stretch. Safety concerns, which are especially acute for women, children, older adults, and members of racial minority groups, mean that outdoor spaces that exist on a map *may not feel accessible in practice*. And for the many Americans working multiple jobs or caring for young children or elderly parents without support, *time is simply not available.*

These are not excuses. They are facts. And they deserve to be treated as facts rather than obstacles to be cheerfully overcome.

## A Problem That Falls Heaviest on Those Who Can Least Afford It

Here is something that should make all of us uncomfortable.

By and large, the people with the least access to nature are the ones who need its benefits the most.

According to a 2020 report from the Center for American Progress called *The Nature Gap*—a comprehensive analysis of nature access across the United States—communities of color are three times more likely than white communities to live in areas with limited access to nature. In the contiguous United States, 74 percent of communities of color face what researchers call a "*nature deficit,*" compared with only 23 percent of white communities. Seventy percent of low-income communities face similar challenges. For low-income communities of color, more than 76 percent of residents live in nature-deprived areas.

***Read those numbers again***. Three out of four people in communities of color in this country. More than seven out of ten people in low-income communities. Living in places where nature—the trees, the parks, the green spaces, the clean air—is *simply not part of their daily environment.*

***This is not an accident.*** Research published in major journals over the past decade has traced the distribution of green space in American cities back to historical policies including redlining, discriminatory zoning, and deliberate disinvestment in lower-income and minority communities. The absence of trees and parks in these neighborhoods isn't a neutral fact of geography. It is the physical legacy of decisions that were made, often explicitly, to concentrate environmental benefits in wealthier and whiter communities.

The research on green space and health equity makes this injustice concrete. A systematic review published in the International Journal of Environmental Research and Public Health found that disadvantaged populations—those with lower incomes and from racial and ethnic minority groups—show the strongest health benefits from green space when they have access to it. In other words, *the people who benefit most from nature are the people who are most systematically denied access to it.* I didn't want this book to be political, but there is no way around it. Politics have determined matters of health and segregation.

One particularly striking study, focused on Philadelphia, found that increasing tree canopy in low-income neighborhoods was associated with a significant narrowing of income-based inequalities in mental health outcomes. Trees—not psychiatric medication, not expensive therapy, not gym memberships—trees. The simplest, most ancient form of nature contact, narrowing health gaps that have persisted for generations.

I want to be clear about what this means. *This isn't just a personal wellness issue. It is a public health and social justice issue.* The benefits we have described in this book—reduced anxiety, lower cortisol, improved mood, better sleep, stronger immune function, and greater social connection—aren't available equally to everyone. They are distributed, like so many health resources in this country, in ways that reflect and reinforce existing inequalities. The really dumbfounding issue here is that if you give people access to green space, trees, or parks, you can decrease the money that has to be spent treating illnesses that wouldn't have arisen if they had had access to those types of environments. How does that make any sense?

Acknowledging that isn't the same as accepting it. People are working to change it, and we'll come back to that. But first, let's talk about what the research says you can do right now, wherever you are and whatever your circumstances.

## The Window That Changes Everything

In 1984, a researcher named **Roger Ulrich** published a study in the journal Science that would go on to become *one of the most cited papers in the field of environmental psychology.*

He examined the recovery records of patients who had undergone the same routine gallbladder surgery at a Pennsylvania hospital. Some of those patients had rooms with windows overlooking a small grove of trees. Others had rooms with windows facing a brick wall. *That was the only difference.*

*The results were striking*. Patients who could see the trees from their hospital beds had shorter hospital stays, needed fewer doses of strong pain medication, received fewer negative nursing notes describing them as upset or in need of encouragement, and had slightly better minor complication rates than the patients looking at the wall. It's amazing how similar it is to the results we found when people had music in their environment, either in the operating room or in their rooms while they recovered from surgery.

A view of trees. Not a forest hike. Not a wilderness retreat. *A view of a few trees through a hospital window.* One major new hospital center, NYU Langone in Manhattan, has taken a version of this architectural feature into the urban environment. Patient rooms in that new hospital on the East River Drive have large windows that give a view of the East River and the skyscrapers surrounding the city. In the morning, the sun rises in the corridors facing east and washes them up with morning sunlight that is incredible in its beauty.

Ulrich's study launched four decades of research into what happens when people can see nature—not be in nature, not walk through nature, just see it. And the findings have been remarkably consistent.

A 2025 analysis published in the journal BioScience by researchers Soga and Gaston reviewed 28 studies on the health effects of viewing nature through windows. The results were clear: viewing nature—from the home, from a hospital room, or from a workplace—was consistently *associated with reduced anxiety and depression symptoms, decreased stress and anger, and improved positive emotions,* including *happiness and life satisfaction*. When the researchers looked specifically at surgical patients, nature views were associated with *faster recovery and reduced pain perception*. The benefits were actually greatest for managed nature like gardens and street trees, probably because those tend to be closer to people's windows than wild landscapes.

Another 2025 study from Texas A&M University, published in the journal HERD, *used virtual reality* to test the effects of different hospital room features on stress recovery and mental clarity. Among the features they tested were *window views of green nature, indoor plants, and green wall décor.* The study found that all of the green elements—individually and in combination—produced measurable improvements in physical relaxation and mental clarity. *Window views of nature produced some of the highest restoration scores*. Buildings that blocked nature views were associated with negative outcomes on every recovery measure.

What does this mean for you, practically? It means that if you cannot easily get outside—if you are recovering from surgery, managing a disability, dealing with a chronic illness, or simply living somewhere that doesn't offer easy outdoor access—the view from your window is not nothing. It is something. It's something the research has measured and confirmed, repeatedly, across decades and continents.

If you have a window that looks out onto trees, a garden, a sky with clouds, even a single tree on a city block: *that is nature contact.*

Imperfect, incomplete, but real and measurable. Look at it. Spend time near it. If you can arrange your workspace or your sitting area to face it, do that.

And if you don't have that kind of window view, we're going to talk about what else you can do.

## Bringing the Outside In

One of the simplest and most researched alternatives to outdoor nature access is also one of the most underestimated: *houseplants.*

The research on indoor plants and mental health has been building for decades, and in recent years it has gotten more specific and more convincing. A 2025 literature review from the University of South Dakota examined ten studies on houseplants and mental health outcomes in people who were stuck indoors for extended periods. The findings were consistent: caring for and being around houseplants was associated with reduced anxiety symptoms, lower stress, and improved mood. The mechanism appears to involve several of the same pathways we've discussed throughout this book—*phytoncides from plant leaves, the visual calming effect of green color and organic shapes, and the psychological benefit of nurturing something living.*

A study of urban adults in China, published in the journal Plants, found that people who spent more time caring for houseplants, who had been caring for plants for longer, and who had more houseplants showed measurably higher levels of mental well-being and mindfulness than those without plants. The effect grew with engagement: the more involved people were in caring for their plants—not just looking at them but watering, repotting, and tending them—the stronger the benefit. I know a veterinarian, in a very large stressful practice, who has found that the Japanese art of raising bonsai trees provides what he needs in terms of de-stressing after a complicated work day. A woman, whose sister has a high-power job in entertainment, raises orchids. Many believe they are too delicate to be raised in a home, but orchids happen to be very hardy plants.

Research on hospital patients has found something similar. The Texas A&M study mentioned earlier found that indoor plants produced significant improvements in physical relaxation and mental clarity, particularly for people experiencing higher levels of acute stress. Potted plants in a room, or plants and flowers on a windowsill, were shown to enhance well-being even for people who had no broader view of a natural landscape.

There are also air quality benefits, though these are often overstated in popular media. The original NASA research on air-purifying plants found that certain species do *absorb volatile organic compounds and other indoor pollutants.* The effect is *real but modest*—you would need a lot of plants to meaningfully clean a room's air. The psychological benefits, however, show up even with a small number of plants.

The most important thing to know about houseplants for mental health is this: *real plants work, and fake ones don't.* Multiple studies have found that artificial plants produce little or none of the psychological benefit of real ones, despite the fact that they are green, too. The living quality of the plant—the fact that it is growing, changing, responding to light and water, and alive—appears to be part of what makes the difference.

The second most important thing: *you don't need a lot of them.* One or two thriving plants produce measurable effects. Location matters—put them somewhere you spend time and *where you can actually see them.*

Some particularly useful plants for indoor mental health benefit, based on ease of care and research support, include **pothos** (nearly impossible to kill and shown to reduce stress), **snake plants** (also very hardy and effective at low light), **peace lilies** (shown to reduce stress hormones and grow well indoors), and **lavender** (its scent has strong anxiety-reducing properties that work even indoors). For anyone without a green thumb, pothos and snake plants are the safest starting point. They survive neglect, thrive in indirect light, and keep producing the benefits. In my elementary school the nun who taught one of our classes in 3rd or 4th grade had a number of large snake plants on the window sills in our classroom. She never seemed to touch them but they grew beautifully.

## The Nature You Hear

We covered sound in depth in Chapter 6, but it's worth returning to it briefly here, because nature sounds are one of the most accessible forms of nature contact for people who cannot get outside.

The research on recorded nature sounds is consistent and promising. Studies have found that listening to birdsong, flowing water, rain, and forest sounds produces measurable reductions in stress hormones, heart rate, and self-reported anxiety—even when the sounds come from a speaker or a phone rather than an actual outdoor environment. The brain processes these sounds through pathways that evolved in outdoor environments, and those pathways *don't appear to fully distinguish between recorded and live sources.*

This means that for someone who is *bedbound, housebound, or living in a noisy urban environment* without access to green space, a good pair of headphones and a nature sounds playlist is *not a consolation prize.* It's a real, evidence-supported intervention.

Apps like *Calm, Insight Timer, and YouTube channels* dedicated to nature soundscapes offer free or low-cost access to high-quality recordings of forests, oceans, rain, rivers, and birdsong. For people dealing with anxiety, these can be *particularly effective in the evening* when the nervous system tends to ramp up rather than wind down. You can also find *free downloadable MP3 files* of calming music or natural sounds on the *Internet Archive*. One file entitled "*Rain Forest, Actual Sounds Of Nature*" is an hour long.

## Virtual Nature: More Than It Sounds

I want to spend some time on *virtual nature*, because the research in this area has moved fast and the results are more significant than most people realize.

For a long time, the assumption was that virtual or digital versions of nature—videos, photographs, VR experiences—were pale substitutes at best. Interesting for entertainment, but not genuinely therapeutic. The emerging research is challenging that assumption.

A systematic review and analysis published in the journal *npj Digital Medicine* in November 2025—one of the most comprehensive analyses of this subject to date—examined 24 studies on the effects of exposure to virtual natural environments on stress, anxiety, and depression in healthy adults. *The results were striking.* Exposure to virtual natural environments produced *large reductions in anxiety.* And the statistical effect of anxiety was gauged by researchers were classified as large, moderate reductions in stress, and moderate reductions in depression. The researchers concluded that virtual nature "*has a positive impact on mental health and can serve as a viable alternative when direct access to natural environments is not feasible.*"

An interesting study published in January 2026 in the Journal of Technology in Behavioral Science took this further by examining what happens with repeated—not just single—virtual nature exposure. Over several weeks, participants who engaged with virtual nature daily showed decreasing levels of both anxious arousal (the kind of anxiety that feels like panic) and anxious apprehension (the kind that feels like worry). *Both types of anxiety responded.* They responded to a video displayed on a screen, which included accompanying natural sounds.

If you want to give someone in a demanding profession or who needs to manage stress and anxiety a great gift, consider either the audio of natural sounds or a video with natural sounds and a natural environment. If they use it regularly, this research suggests they will benefit, and their physical and mental health can be positively affected as well.

The clinical applications are being taken seriously. A pilot study published in January 2026 tested a *virtual reality forest therapy program* with 16 psychiatric inpatients—people hospitalized for serious mental health conditions. The patients went through four immersive VR sessions simulating forest environments. The results showed statistically significant improvements in depression, anxiety, stress, and overall well-being. Physiological measures—heart rate variability and electrodermal activity, which track how the nervous system is actually responding—confirmed the improvements weren't just self-reported. The patients' bodies were responding to the virtual forest the way they might respond to a real one.

I've worked in psychiatric hospitals and I know they can be very stressful for staff and patients alike. Patients don't usually have much access to outside areas, so this type of therapy would be incredibly helpful for everyone. Some patients only get outside of locked wards two or maybe three times a day and that's only if there's enough staff and it's safe. Going outside also means 15 to 20 minutes—maybe a half hour, but that's it. It's probably as close to solitary confinement as you can get outside of a prison.

This doesn't mean virtual nature is equivalent to real outdoor time or that it should replace outdoor access for people who have it. The research is clear that real nature produces stronger effects. But for someone who genuinely cannot get outside—a person with severe mobility limitations, someone recovering from a major surgery, someone living in a situation that makes outdoor access impossible—virtual nature is not nothing. It is something the nervous system measurably responds to.

The most accessible form of this is simply watching nature videos on a television or computer screen. YouTube has an enormous library of high-quality nature footage—forests, oceans, meadows, mountains—and channels like Nature Relaxation Films provide hours of footage specifically designed to be calming. For people with access to a VR headset, immersive nature experiences produce even stronger effects, and the technology has become significantly more affordable recently.

One caution worth naming: *some people experience motion sickness or disorientation with VR*, particularly if they are older or have vestibular conditions. Start with shorter sessions and flat or slowly moving footage rather than immersive action-based experiences.

## Green Design: The Spaces You Live In

For people who have some choice over their living or working environment—which is not everyone, and I recognize that—the research on biophilic design offers practical guidance about how to bring more nature into indoor spaces.

Biophilic design is the practice of incorporating natural elements into built environments. It ranges from simple choices like adding plants and using natural materials to larger architectural decisions like *installing atriums, green walls, and windows designed to maximize light and nature views.* In fact there is a whole new discipline in architecture called *biophilic architecture*. Do a search on the Internet and you may be amazed at the things they are doing to building design to incorporate nature in all its forms today. The principle behind it is the same one we've discussed throughout this book: the human nervous system evolved in natural environments, and it responds positively to the features of those environments even when they're recreated indoors.

The research on biophilic design in workplaces and healthcare settings is well-established. A 2021 study found that offices with integrated greenery showed a *26 percent increase in cognitive performance* and a *15 percent decrease in sick days*. Studies on hospital design consistently find that patients in rooms with natural light, nature views, and indoor plants recover faster, use less pain medication, and report higher satisfaction with their care.

For someone working from home or spending a lot of time in one indoor space, some of the most impactful changes are also the simplest: moving a desk or a chair near a window, adding plants, choosing natural materials over synthetic ones, and using lighting that mimics natural light cycles (warmer and dimmer in the evening, brighter and cooler in the morning).

Natural textures—wood, stone, cotton, and linen—appear to have calming effects that synthetic materials don't. This change is a small thing, but small things accumulate.

Nature-inspired artwork is worth mentioning here. Multiple studies have found that *looking at photographs and paintings of natural landscapes* produces stress-reducing effects, though they are smaller than those produced by real views or real nature contact. For someone without access to a window with a nature view, a large, high-quality photograph or painting of a forest, coastline, or meadow on the wall of a room where they spend time is a genuine, evidence-supported option.

## What You Can Do Right Now: A Practical Guide

All of the research in this chapter points toward the same practical conclusion: the benefits of nature exist on a spectrum, and almost everyone can access some point on that spectrum, even if they can't access the full outdoor experience this book has focused on.

Here is a practical framework, organized from the most accessible to the more involved.

**If you can't get outside at all:**

1. Sit near a window with a view of any natural element—a tree, the sky, or a garden. *Spend at least ten minutes a day with that view.*

2. Add one or two real, living houseplants to the space where you spend the most time. Pothos and snake plants are the easiest starting point. *Put them where you can see them.*

3. Listen to recorded nature sounds for twenty to thirty minutes a day, especially in the evening. *Use headphones for a stronger effect.*

4. *Watch high-quality nature videos on a screen*—real footage of forests, oceans, or open landscapes, not just relaxation music with nature images. YouTube and streaming services have extensive options.

5. *Use natural light when possible.* Open blinds and curtains during daylight hours, even if you can't go outside.

***If you can get outside occasionally but not easily:***

Even five minutes outside matters. The research on "doses" of nature consistently finds that short exposures produce real effects—effects that are not zero just because they're brief.

*Sit outside* rather than walk if walking is difficult. A chair on a porch, a bench near your building, or even an open window you can lean out of slightly puts you in contact with outdoor air, outdoor light, and outdoor sound in ways that have measurable effects.

*Target early morning* or late afternoon outdoor time to maximize sunlight exposure while avoiding peak heat. These are also the times when birdsong is typically most active.

If weather or safety is a barrier, look for alternatives: covered porches, enclosed courtyards, indoor atriums or botanical gardens in your city, shopping malls with significant natural light and planted areas.

If your neighborhood lacks green space, identify the nearest park—even a small one—and *plan occasional visits* rather than daily ones. Even infrequent contact with green space has been shown to produce lasting effects on mood and stress.

***If you're supporting someone else who can't get outside:***

*Bring nature to them.* Fresh flowers, potted plants, and natural materials make a real difference in the environment of someone who is housebound or hospitalized.

*Set up a screen near their bed or chair* with nature videos or a window-facing webcam of an outdoor space. Nature sounds on a portable speaker can provide auditory contact with natural environments around the clock.

If you are a caregiver or healthcare provider, *advocate for natural light, window views, and indoor plants* in the care settings where you work. The research supports these as genuine health interventions, not decorative extras. I remember when I was consulting at a nursing home. One day, as I talked to a woman whose bed was next to a window, I noticed that an occasional bird would come by and she would be thrilled. It sparked an idea for me.

I told management at that facility that I believed they should put *bird feeders in the trees near patients' windows.* They did. The birds came incredibly fast, and the patients were so enlivened. They talked about which birds came, when they came, and how many came. It was a whole new environment in that place. Unfortunately, so many birds came that the maintenance staff began to complain about having to refill the feeders too many times during the day. They had to put some restrictions on them but the patients still benefited when the feeders were filled and the birds came. I never saw so many smiling faces that previously were absolutely bland.

## The Larger Picture

I want to end this chapter by saying something that goes beyond the individual practical tips.

The barriers we've discussed in this chapter—*disability, chronic illness, urban density, poverty, racism in the built environment*—are not personal problems to be solved by individual creativity and willpower. *They are structural problems that require structural responses.*

Cities that invest in green space are cities that are investing in public health. When Milwaukee transforms a parking lot into a community garden, when Fort Collins creates a network of accessible open spaces, when Philadelphia plants trees in low-income neighborhoods and watches the mental health gap narrow as a result—these are not soft amenity projects. *These are health interventions with a measurable return.*

Healthcare systems that *prescribe nature*—that give patients an actual written prescription to spend time in a park, backed by referrals to local programs that support that access—are practicing *evidence-based medicine*. The NaturRx and ParkRx movements, now active in cities across the country, are taking exactly this approach. Doctors writing prescriptions. Not for pills. For parks.

Architects and builders who design living walls, atriums, window views, and natural materials into hospitals, schools, offices, and apartment buildings are not indulging aesthetic preferences. They are building environments that measurably improve the health of the people who spend time in them.

None of this excuses individuals from taking what action they can within their own lives and circumstances. The tips in this chapter are real and the research behind them is solid. If you can't get to a forest, a houseplant is not nothing. A window view is not nothing. A nature video is not nothing.

But the people who face the most severe barriers to nature access are not going to solve this problem one houseplant at a time. They need—and deserve—the same access to what amounts to a fundamental health resource that wealthier and whiter communities take for granted.

*Nature is not a luxury*. It is a health necessity. And the research in this chapter, taken together, makes a clear and urgent case that access to it should be treated like any other health resource: something that everyone deserves, and something we should work—together, systematically—to ensure it is available to everyone who needs it.

Until then, do what you can with what you have. A window. A plant. A pair of headphones and ten minutes of birdsong. The benefits are real, even when they are partial. Even when the door won't open all the way.

*Start there. And keep pushing for the door to open wider.*

## What's Coming Next

We've now spent eight chapters exploring how the outdoor environment—and when necessary, indoor versions of it—shapes your mental and physical health. In Chapter 9, we're going to bring everything together with a focus on one of the most practical questions readers ask: *How do I actually make this a habit?*

Knowing that outdoor time is good for you isn't the same as *doing it consistently*. Chapter 9 will look at the behavioral science of *habit formation* and apply it specifically to the challenge of building a sustainable relationship with nature—one that holds up against the real pressures of a busy life, bad weather, low motivation, and the endless competing demands on your attention.

*Because the research only matters if you actually use it.*

## CHAPTER 8 REFERENCES

Bratman, G. N., et al. (2019). Nature and mental health: An ecosystem service perspective. Science Advances, 5(7), eaax0903. https://doi.org/10.1126/sciadv.aax0903

Browning, M. H. E. M., et al. (2020). Can simulated nature support mental health? Comparing short, single doses of 360-degree nature videos in virtual reality with the outdoors. Frontiers in Psychology, 11, 567200. https://doi.org/10.3389/fpsyg.2020.567200

Center for American Progress. (2020). The nature gap: Confronting racial and economic disparities in the destruction and protection of nature in America. https://www.americanprogress.org/article/the-nature-gap/

Hui, X., et al. (2025). Virtual nature, real relief: How exposure to virtual natural environments reduces anxiety, stress, and depression in healthy adults. npj Digital Medicine, 8, 679. https://doi.org/10.1038/s41746-025-02057-4

Jiayu He, Yuanning Guo, Jiamin Chen, Jinhua Xu, Xiaohua Zhu. Exploring the correlation between UVB sensitivity and SLE activity: Insights into UVB-driven pathogenesis in lupus erythematosus, Journal of Autoimmunity, Volume 153, 2025, 103393, ISSN 0896-8411, https://doi.org/10.1016/j.jaut.2025.103393. (https://www.sciencedirect.com/science/article/pii/S0896841125000381).

Kondo, M. C., et al. (2018). Urban green space and its impact on human health. International Journal of Environmental Research and Public Health, 15(3), 445. https://doi.org/10.3390/ijerph15030445

Mitchell, R., & Popham, F. (2008). Effect of exposure to natural environment on health inequalities: An observational population study. The Lancet, 372(9650), 1655–1660. https://doi.org/10.1016/S0140-6736(08)61689-X

Rigolon, A., Browning, M., McAnirlin, O., & Yoon, H. V. (2021). Green space and health equity: A systematic review on the potential of green space to reduce health disparities. International Journal of Environmental Research and Public Health, 18(5), 2563. https://doi.org/10.3390/ijerph18052563

Soga, M., & Gaston, K. J. (2025). Health benefits of viewing nature through windows: A meta-analysis. BioScience, 75(8), 628–640. https://doi.org/10.1093/biosci/biaf059

South, E. C., et al. (2018). Effect of greening vacant land on mental health of community-dwelling adults: A cluster randomized trial.

JAMA Network Open, 1(3), e180298. https://doi.org/10.1001/jamanetworkopen.2018.0298

Suess, C., & Maddock, J. (2025). Understanding the influence of window views, plantscapes, and green décor in virtual reality hospital rooms on simulated acute-care patients' stress recovery and relaxation responses. HERD: Health Environments Research & Design Journal, 18(3), 165–183. https://doi.org/10.1177/19375867251344626

Umucu, E., et al. (2025). Health inequities among persons with disabilities: A global scoping review. Frontiers in Public Health, 13, 1538519. https://doi.org/10.3389/fpubh.2025.1538519

Ulrich, R. S. (1984). View through a window may influence recovery from surgery. Science, 224(4647), 420–421. https://doi.org/10.1126/science.6143402

Vo, D., et al. (2026). The impact of virtual reality-based forest therapy in psychiatric inpatient care: A pilot study. Advances in Mental Health, online first. https://doi.org/10.1080/18387357.2026.2615679

White, M. P., et al. (2018). A prescription for "nature"—The potential of using virtual nature in therapeutics. Neuropsychiatric Disease and Treatment, 14, 3001–3013. https://doi.org/10.2147/NDT.S179038

Ye, X., et al. (2024). Reduction in socioeconomic inequalities in self-reported mental health conditions with increasing greenspace exposure. PMC Article, PMID 38851973. https://pmc.ncbi.nlm.nih.gov/articles/PMC11151689/

# Chapter 9: Making It Stick: The Behavioral Science of Building an Outdoor Habit That Lasts

Here is something I have noticed after many years of working with people on behavior change: *knowing what to do is almost never the problem.*

By the time you have gotten to this chapter, you know what the research says. You know that spending time outside reduces stress hormones, lifts mood, quiets the mind, and builds *the kind of mental resilience that no pill or app can fully replicate*. You have read the studies. You understand the biology.

But if you're honest, you've probably known something was good for you and still didn't do it consistently. *That isn't a personal failing. It is a description of how human brains work.* If you had good intentions and you weren't following through on them, don't beat yourself up. There are things you can do, and there are reasons you don't do them. The secret lies in understanding habits and how to best use them to your advantage. Most of the time we're told that habits are things we should learn to break. Yet here I'm advocating for you to learn how to use habits and not lose them. Are you with me?

*Habits are not built on knowledge.* They are *not built on motivation, either*. Motivation is a feeling, and feelings rise and fall with your sleep quality, your stress level, the weather, and whether your commute was difficult. **Motivation can't be counted on**. Toss that one aside. The research on this is clear and unambiguous: if getting outside is *something you only do when you feel like it*, you won't do it enough to matter.

What the science tells us about building any lasting behavior is that you have to *stop relying on feeling like it* and ***start relying on structure***. That's what this chapter is about.

## The 21-Day Myth and What Actually Happens in Your Brain

Most people have heard that it *takes 21 days to form a habit.* That number has been repeated so many times in self-help books and wellness articles that it has taken on the quality of fact. **It's not a fact.** *It is a misquote from a 1960 book by a* ***plastic surgeon***, and it was *never a scientific finding* to begin with. It's beginning to sound like those 10,000 steps isn't it? It's a catchy book title but it's nothing more. Again, toss that one aside or in the bin. There's no benefit in holding on to myths or falsehoods that someone manufactured to make themselves sound smart.

Too many people assign the title of "expert" to themselves with no support for that honorific. But once the press releases go out and the statements begin to sound so seductive and are repeated time and time again in all those clickbait headlines, it's almost impossible to stop them. They become ingrained in our culture even though *they are myths that someone made up* to make themselves look more than they really are. Personal puffery has led to myths. An example where this happened in a psychology experiment about stress called " *The Executive Monkey Experiment.*" People continue to say it was the executive monkey that was at risk. Wrong. Read up on it in the references at the end of this section.

Here is what the science actually says. A major 2025 systematic review from the University of South Australia—*one of the most comprehensive analyses of habit formation ever conducted*—looked at data from more than 2,600 people across 20 studies. The average time it took a new behavior to become genuinely automatic was **around *two months***. And the range was enormous: *some habits formed in as little as four days, while others took nearly a year.* Considering how long or short the time is for forming a habit last, it's pretty incredible and variable.

What determined the difference? *Simplicity, consistency, and context*. Simple behaviors *tied to a stable daily context* and repeated at the same time and place formed faster. Complex behaviors with inconsistent cues took much longer. The researchers also found something useful and encouraging: *missing a day here and there didn't derail the process.* Habit formation is gradual, not fragile.

What is happening in your brain during this process? When you first try a new behavior, your prefrontal cortex is running the show. It is the part of the brain *responsible for conscious decision-making*, and it takes real energy to use it. That's why new habits feel like work. But as you repeat the behavior in consistent conditions, a deeper brain structure called *the basal ganglia* starts to take over. That bit of the brain *specializes in storing automatic routines*—patterns so well-worn *they no longer require conscious thought*. I suppose you could say that tying your shoelaces would be something that had been assigned to this brain area. After learning to tie your shoelaces, you do it almost automatically in the future. Once your outdoor habit reaches that stage, you don't decide to go outside. You just go. That transition from conscious effort to automatic behavior is the essence of what habit formation actually is.

## Dr. Wood's Key Insight: Context, Not Willpower

Wendy Wood, a social psychologist at the University of Southern California, has spent decades studying how habits form and why they stick. In a January 2026 interview with the American Psychological Association, she said something worth reading twice: ***habits do not develop through motivation***. They develop through repeated experience in a stable context that yields a reward. We can say that's a formula for success for habit formation.

That word *context* is the one to hold onto. The research shows consistently that people who form durable habits are *not more motivated* or more disciplined than people who fail. They are *people who have designed their environment to make the behavior easy and unavoidable*. They reduced the friction between wanting to do something and actually doing it.

What does that mean for getting outside? It means that the person who *puts their walking shoes by the door every night* is more likely to walk in the morning than the person who has to find them. The person who has an *outdoor lunch location already chosen* is more likely to eat outside than the person who has to decide in the moment. The person who walks past a park on the way to the coffee shop is more likely to stop than the person who has to go out of their way.

You aren't battling laziness. **You are designing context**. Those are completely different things, and only one of them actually works.

## The 120-Minute Target and How to Reach It

The most solid number in all the outdoor health research is *120 minutes per week*. A major study published in Scientific Reports found that people who spent at least two hours a week in natural outdoor settings reported significantly better health and well-being than those who spent less—and this finding held regardless of how they distributed that time across the week. We always have to consider self-report measures as perhaps not as robust as measures we would get from biological material or measurements such as blood pressure, body heat, whatever.

Two hours a week. That is about *17 minutes per day*. Or three 40-minute outings. Or two full hours spread out, however it fits your life.

The reason this number matters is that *it gives you a target* that is both meaningful and achievable. You're not being asked to move to the countryside or overhaul your entire schedule. You are being asked to find 120 minutes somewhere in a 168-hour week.

The behavioral research supports something called the Minimal Viable Habit—the smallest version of a new behavior that still produces real benefit. For outdoor time, that is around *20 minutes at a go*. Twenty minutes has been shown in multiple studies to *measurably reduce cortisol, improve mood, and restore directed attention.* It's not nothing. And it is achievable even on difficult days. Can you find twenty minutes in your day where you can spend it outdoors? I think you can.

**Start there.** Not with an hour-long nature walk that requires planning and perfect weather. Start with *20 minutes three times a week* and build from that foundation. You might want to put a small chart on your refrigerator (or someplace you're sure to see it) and each day indicate how close you've come to your target time outside. A simple graph would be helpful, too.

## Anchor Habits: Attaching the New to the Old

One of the most reliable techniques in behavioral science is called *habit stacking, or anchoring*. It's a technique that is also used in learning anything that might be complex such as math or reading. The idea is simple: you attach the new behavior you want to build onto an existing behavior that already happens automatically.

You already go outside to get to your car in the morning. You already eat lunch. You already walk to a meeting sometimes. You already take the dog out. These are automatic behaviors, and they are *strong enough to carry a new behavior attached to them.*

The formula is straightforward: ***after I do X, I will do Y***. After I drop the kids at school, I will walk for twenty minutes before getting back in the car. After I eat lunch, I will spend fifteen minutes outside before returning to my desk. After I take the dog out in the morning, I will stay outside an extra ten minutes sit quietly.

The anchor doesn't have to be complicated. It just has to be something you already do without thinking. The new behavior borrows the existing behavior's automatic quality. Over time, the combination becomes *a single automatic sequence*, and the outdoor portion starts to feel as natural as the anchor that preceded it.

## Reducing Friction: Making It Easier to Go Than to Stay

*Every obstacle* between you and the habit *is a piece of frictio*n, and friction is the enemy of consistency. Research in behavioral economics consistently shows that small increases in friction can dramatically reduce how often people do something, even when they want to do it.

The reverse is also true. *Every time you make a behavior slightly easier, slightly more convenient, slightly more automatic, you increase the odds that it happens.* This is not about motivation. It is about **design**.

Think through what makes getting outside harder than it needs to be. If it's clothing or shoes, keep them accessible. If it's weather uncertainty, identify covered or sheltered outdoor spots in advance. If it's feeling like you need a plan or a destination, let yourself just walk without one. If it's feeling unsafe, identify routes you trust, or reach out to someone who can join you.

One practical approach: *identify one outdoor spot within ten minutes of where you spend most of your time*. It doesn't need to be impressive. A park bench. A tree-lined block. A parking lot with a bit of green at the edge. Something you can reach quickly, without a car, without planning, and without preparation. That spot is your default. When in doubt, you go there.

## Implementation Intentions: Planning Around the Obstacles

One of the most well-tested strategies in behavior change research is called an *implementation intention*, which is a fancy name for *a very practical technique*. A plain-language description is ***if-then planning***. You anticipate the specific obstacle that will come up and decide in advance how you will handle it.

Research by psychologist Peter Gollwitzer, published in the American Psychologist, found that people who formed implementation intentions were two to three times more likely to follow through on their intentions than people who only formed goals. The difference wasn't motivation. It was specificity.

Here is how it works for outdoor time: instead of deciding that you will try to get outside more, you decide that if it's raining when you normally go out, then you will put on a rain jacket and go anyway, or you will use the covered walkway by the library instead. If you miss your morning walk, then you will take a 15-minute outdoor break at noon instead. If you feel too tired to go out, then you will tell yourself you only have to go for five minutes—and you can come back if you still want to after five minutes. *Almost no one comes back after five minutes.*

The key is that you are making these decisions when you are calm and clear-headed, not in the moment when you are tired or busy or tempted to skip. Pre-decided responses to predictable obstacles take the decision out of the moment. And the moment is exactly where willpower runs out.

## The Never Miss Two Rule

Here is the *only rule you need for dealing* **with** the inevitable days when you miss your outdoor time: **never miss two in a row.**

Missing once doesn't break a habit. The University of South Australia research confirmed this—occasional lapses don't undo the habit formation process. *What breaks habits is missing multiple times in succession*, because each missed day makes the next one slightly easier to miss until the behavior has quietly disappeared from your life.

The **never-miss-two rule** gives you both forgiveness and a limit. You are allowed to miss a day. Life is complicated, and perfect consistency isn't the goal. The goal is getting back out the next day. One missed day is a pause. Two missed days is the beginning of a pattern. Three is the habit unraveling.

This rule is easier to apply than it sounds because it reframes the day after a miss as critically important—as the day that protects the whole thing. Even if you only go out for ten minutes the day after you missed, *you have kept the chain alive.* That matters more than the duration. Go for those 10 minutes if you missed the day before. Don't let that two-day span mean you've just broken an important chain in your behavior and in helping yourself. Be your best friend and do it.

## Tracking: The Simple Kind That Works

Research has consistently found that tracking habits increases follow-through. But there is an important nuance: *simple tracking works better* than complicated tracking, especially during the habit formation phase.

A 2025 study found that people using simple binary tracking—*did I do it today, yes or* no?—maintained new habits 27 percent longer than people using detailed tracking systems. *The detail gets in the way.* Simple is better. The question you need to answer every day is not how long, how far, or how many steps. It is: *did I go outside today?* This is where we get away from our technologically oriented culture and return to the simpler things in life. It's a yes or no and that's it.

Mark a calendar. Put a check on a piece of paper. Keep it visible. Keep it honest. The visual record of consistency becomes its own motivation—most people don't want to break a streak—and the visibility of the record keeps the habit in your awareness rather than letting it drift out of your attention.

## Your 12-Week Starting Framework

Here is a practical structure to build your outdoor habit *over the first three months,* based on what the behavioral research supports. There is no absolute rule here, and *this is not a rigid format* that anyone needs to follow. If you have any concerns, please discuss them with a healthcare professional or a trusted friend.

**Weeks one and two**: go outside once a day for at least *20 minutes.* Don't worry about where you go or what you do. The only goal is to get your body outside every day and to *attach the outing to an anchor behavior that already exists in your routine.*

**Weeks three through six**: *add a second daily outing* when possible—morning and noon, or noon and after dinner. Your goal is still simple: accumulate time outside. *Identify your if-then responses for the obstacles* you have already encountered. Start tracking with a simple calendar.

**Weeks seven through twelve**: you are *aiming for your 120-minute weekly target.* Some days will be longer, some shorter. The **never-miss-two rule** is your safety net. By week twelve, research suggests you should begin to feel the difference between days you went outside and days you didn't—and that difference becomes its own motivation. I once worked with a therapist whose husband went jogging every day when he came home. One day he couldn't go jogging because it was raining so heavily and he told her he felt so depressed after not jogging. He really missed it. What he was missing was the physiological surge that being outside and jogging had been giving him. For him it was like an addiction in the best way.

**After week twelve**, you aren't done building the habit. *You are done building it deliberately*. From here, the goal is consistency, not effort. The basal ganglia have taken over. You have stopped deciding to go outside and *started just going.*

## When You Need More Than a Habit

It would be dishonest to end this chapter without saying clearly: outdoor time is a powerful tool, *but it's not a substitute for professional mental health care when that care is needed.*

If you are experiencing symptoms of ***serious depression, anxiety, trauma, or any other mental health condition***, please work with a qualified professional. The research in this book supports *outdoor* *time as a complement to treatment*—something that makes therapy and other interventions more effective, *not something that replaces them.*

The habit you are building here serves as a foundation. It makes everything else easier. But foundations aren't the whole structure, and if you need more support, *asking for it isn't a failure.* It is *exactly the right thing to do.*

*Now go outside.*

## References

Cleveland Clinic. (2024, June 18). Everything you need to know about habit stacking for self-improvement. Cleveland Clinic Health Essentials. https://health.clevelandclinic.org/habit-stacking

Fournier, M., et al. (2017). Effects of a text-messaging intervention on physical activity: A meta-analysis. Behavioral Medicine, 43(4), 263–274. https://doi.org/10.1080/08964289.2016.1222347

Gardner, B., Rebar, A. L., & Lally, P. (2020). A matter of habit: Recognizing the multiple roles of habit in health behavior. British Journal of General Practice, 70(699), 514–515. https://doi.org/10.3399/bjgp20X712597

Gollwitzer, P. M. (1999). Implementation intentions: Strong effects of simple plans. American Psychologist, 54(7), 493–503. https://doi.org/10.1037/0003-066X.54.7.493

Harvey, A. G., & Gumport, N. B. (2022). Applying the science of habit formation to evidence-based psychological treatments for mental illness. Perspectives on Psychological Science, 17(2), 572–589. https://doi.org/10.1177/1745691621995752

Inglis-Arkell, E. (2014, October 8). The problem with the famously godawful executive monkey study. Gizmodo. https://gizmodo.com/the-problem-with-the-famously-godawful-executive-monkey-1643699082

Lally, P., van Jaarsveld, C. H. M., Potts, H. W. W., & Wardle, J. (2010). How are habits formed: Modeling habit formation in the real world. European Journal of Social Psychology, 40(6), 998–1009. https://doi.org/10.1002/ejsp.674

Milkman, K. L. (2021). How to change: The science of getting from where you are to where you want to be. Portfolio/Penguin.

Singh B, Murphy A, Maher C, Smith AE. Time to Form a Habit: A Systematic Review and Meta-Analysis of Health Behaviour Habit Formation and Its Determinants. Healthcare (Basel). 2024 Dec 9;12(23):2488. doi: 10.3390/healthcare12232488. PMID: 39685110; PMCID: PMC11641623.

Soga, M., et al. (2025). A systematic review and meta-analysis on the effect of nature exposure dose on adults with mental illness. PMC11851813. https://pmc.ncbi.nlm.nih.gov/articles/PMC11851813/

Tyrvainen, L., et al. (2014). The influence of urban green environments on stress relief measures: A field experiment. Journal of Environmental Psychology, 38, 1–9. https://doi.org/10.1016/j.jenvp.2013.12.005

White, M. P., Alcock, I., Grellier, J., Wheeler, B. W., Hartig, T., Warber, S. L., Bone, A., Depledge, M. H., & Fleming, L. E. (2019). Spending at least 120 minutes a week in nature is associated with good health and well-being. Scientific Reports, 9(1), 7730. https://doi.org/10.1038/s41598-019-44097-3

Wood, W. (2026, January). Wendy Wood helps people apply the science of habits in everyday life. Monitor on Psychology,

57(1). https://www.apa.org/monitor/2026/01-02/wendy-wood-habits-behavior-change

Wood, W., & Neal, D. T. (2016). Healthy through habit: Interventions for initiating and maintaining health behavior change. Behavioral Science & Policy, 2(1), 71–83. https://doi.org/10.1353/bsp.2016.0008

# Chapter 10: Your Plan, Your Future, Our World: Putting Everything Together

You have read nine chapters of science. You understand the research. And somewhere in there, I hope something shifted—not just in your thinking, but in *the way you see the ordinary world outside your door.*

That is what happened to me. I didn't start out as someone who believed in the healing power of nature. I was a skeptic, trained in the empirical tradition of academic psychology, trained to trust what could be measured and replicated and published in peer-reviewed journals. And what the peer-reviewed journals told me, the more I dug into this literature, was that being outside is one of the most effective and most underused mental health interventions we have.

I started going outside more deliberately. Not dramatically—no week-long wilderness retreats, no dramatic transformation. Just more intentionally. A morning walk before turning on any screens. Lunch outside when the weather allowed. Choosing to sit in a park rather than a coffee shop when I needed to think through something difficult. Small choices, repeated often enough to become automatic.

The changes were subtle at first, and then they were not subtle at all. My thinking was clearer. The low-grade tension that I had accepted as a normal part of adult professional life eased up. I slept better. I was more present with the people around me. And I started paying attention to what the research was consistently showing for the people I worked with as well.

The science gave me permission to do something I had been dismissing as indulgent. It turned out the science was right.

## What This Book Taught You: The Core Principles

Before you step into your own plan, let's bring the core principles together.

**First**, your brain was shaped by the natural world. The human nervous system didn't evolve in offices, apartment buildings, or under fluorescent lights. It evolved in complex outdoor environments full of sensory information—scent, sound, movement, light, water, and biological diversity. When you return to those environments, even briefly, you are giving your brain and body the conditions they were designed to operate in. The research doesn't just show correlation; it shows mechanisms. Cortisol drops. Serotonin rises. The amygdala quiets. Attention restores. These are not metaphors. *They are measurable biological events.*

**Second**: the dose matters, but the threshold is low. You don't need to become a wilderness adventurer to get these benefits. The research points to 120 minutes per week as a meaningful threshold—and most of those studies are looking at ordinary parks, backyards, tree-lined streets, and waterfront paths. Twenty minutes at a time. Three or four times a week. The bar is low enough for almost anyone, in almost any setting, to clear it.

**Third**: different outdoor environments offer different benefits. Forests activate the body's *relaxation response* and lower blood pressure. Water environments quiet the default mode network—that *mental chatter of rumination and worry*. Natural soundscapes *restore directed attention.* Morning sunlight *resets the biological clock* and drives serotonin. Exercise in green settings produces *mood effects that indoor exercise doesn't replicate*. Knowing what different environments offer lets you match your outdoor time to what you actually need.

**Fourth**: outdoor time is *a complement, not a replacement*. If you are managing a mental health condition, this isn't a reason to abandon your treatment plan. The evidence supports outdoor time as something that *makes everything else work better*—therapy, medication, sleep hygiene, social connection. It belongs in the toolkit, alongside those things, *not instead of them.*

**Fifth**: *the habit has to stick to matter.* One good weekend in nature resets you temporarily. Regular outdoor time, built into your daily structure and maintained through the behavioral strategies in Chapter 9, changes you over time. The research on long-term *nature exposure shows cumulative benefits*—a lower baseline of stress, a more resilient mood, a better-regulated nervous system. Those changes are available to you. But only if you keep going out.

## Your Starting Point

Where you start depends entirely on where you are right now. *And where you are right now is fine.* You don't need to be in good shape. You don't need to live near impressive natural scenery. You don't need to identify as an outdoor person.

If you are sedentary and your mental health is struggling, your starting point might be a ten-minute walk around the block after dinner. That isn't a compromise. *That is a real starting point with real benefits.* The research on brief outdoor exposures shows that ten to twenty minutes is enough to produce measurable changes in stress hormones and mood. You're not starting too small. *You are starting.*

If you have physical limitations, your starting point might be sitting on a porch, opening a window, or spending time in a garden. The evidence from Chapter 8 is clear: even passive nature contact—looking at trees through a window, sitting outside without moving, hearing water—produces benefits. The goal is contact, not performance.

If you live in a dense urban environment, your starting point is *whatever green or blue space is within reasonable reach.* A city park. A river path. A community garden. A block with mature trees. Urban green spaces deliver real benefits—smaller than wilderness settings, but real and measurable. *Start with what you have.* Don't bemoan what you don't have and remember to see what you do have.

If you are already fairly active outdoors, your starting point is becoming more intentional. The research shows that paying deliberate attention to your natural surroundings—noticing what you smell, what you hear, how the light is falling—increases the restorative benefit beyond what you get from moving through an outdoor environment on autopilot. You have been getting some of the benefit. *You can get more.*

## The World Is Moving Toward You

Something remarkable has been happening in medicine and public health over the last decade. The idea that time in nature is a legitimate health intervention—something that can and should be prescribed, tracked, and integrated into mainstream healthcare—has gone from a fringe position to an established and growing movement.

In Canada, PaRx—the national nature prescription program backed by the Canadian Medical Association and endorsed by more than 100 major health organizations—has now distributed over a million nature prescriptions to Canadians. The prescription is simple: *spend at least two hours a week outdoors, 20 minutes at a time.* Doctors write it like any other prescription. Patients fill it like any other treatment.

In the United States, Park Rx America maintains a searchable database of parks and public lands across the country, specifically to connect healthcare providers with nature access points for their patients. More than 100 park prescription programs operate across the US, and the number grows every year.

At NC State University, the campus health system began offering nature prescriptions to students in early 2026. At institutions across Norway, Japan, and the United Kingdom, *green prescriptions have been integrated into standard care pathways.* The World Health Organization has formally recognized nature-based interventions as part of a comprehensive approach to public mental health.

The medical establishment has looked at this evidence and reached the same conclusion that the research has been pointing toward for decades: *going outside is medicine.* You are not pursuing some alternative health trend. You are doing exactly what the science—and now the formal institutions of healthcare—recommend.

## The Bigger Picture: You and the Natural World

There is one more thing I want to say before this book closes, and it is the thing that took me the longest to see clearly.

The research on nature and mental health isn't just about what nature does for you. It is also about what happens to people who spend time in nature: *they start to care more about protecting it.*

This is not a morality argument. It is an empirical one. Miles Richardson's research on nature connectedness consistently finds that people who develop a relationship with the natural world—who feel genuinely connected to it, who notice it, who spend time in it—are more likely to take actions to protect it. *The relationship goes both ways. Nature heals you. And when you are healed by something, you want to keep it.*

This matters because the natural environments that make you healthier are under significant pressure. A 2025 study in Nature Climate Change found that the health costs attributable to climate change are already large and growing. Green spaces in urban areas face development pressure. Noise and light pollution are expanding. Access to nature remains profoundly unequal, with lower-income communities and communities of color consistently showing less access to quality green space.

You cannot individually solve those problems. But you can be part of the constituency that takes them seriously. People who spend time in nature vote for parks. They support conservation. They make different choices about the spaces they create and maintain. *The personal health case and the environmental case are not separate arguments.* They converge in the same place: **the value of the living world.**

E.O. Wilson called it biophilia—the deep, evolved human need for connection with other living things. He believed it was not just a preference but a biological necessity, woven into us by millions of years of evolution in complex natural environments. If he was right, then the modern epidemic of disconnection from nature is not just a health crisis. It is a loss of something fundamental to what we are.

Getting outside is a small act of reclaiming it.

## The Last Thing I Want to Tell You

When I started this book, I thought I was writing about research. And I was. But somewhere along the way, I realized I was also writing about something I had lived. The science gave me the language, but the experience gave me the conviction.

I know what it feels like to believe that indoor, sedentary, screen-mediated life is just what adult life is. I know what it feels like to be too busy, too tired, too stressed to add one more thing into my life. I know what it feels like to be skeptical of anything that sounds too simple or too good.

I also know what it feels like on the other side of that. When going outside became something I did every day, not because I had to but because I noticed what happened when I didn't. When the air smelled like rain and I knew, in some wordless way, what that smell was doing in my brain. When I sat by water and felt something unclench in my chest that I hadn't even known was clenched.

*The research is real. The benefits are real. And they are available to you, wherever you are, with whatever you have access to, starting today.*

You already know what to do.

**Get out!**

## References

BC Parks Foundation. (2025). PaRx: A nature prescription program. https://www.bcparksfoundation.ca/parx/

Carlson, C. J., Mitchell, D., Gibb, R., et al. (2025). Health losses attributed to anthropogenic climate change. Nature Climate Change, 15, 1052–1055. https://doi.org/10.1038/s41558-025-02399-7

Coventry, P., et al. (2021). Nature-based outdoor activities for mental and physical health: Systematic review and meta-analysis. SSM — Population Health, 16, 100934. https://doi.org/10.1016/j.ssmph.2021.100934

Epel, E., et al. (2025). Effects of a novel psychosocial climate resilience course on climate distress, self-efficacy, and mental health in young adults. Sustainability, 17, 3139. https://doi.org/10.3390/su17073139

Fontana, K. (2026, March 13). Campus health now offering nature prescriptions. NC State Global One Health Academy. https://provost.ncsu.edu/global-one-health-academy/2026/03/13/campus-health-now-offering-nature-prescriptions/

Frumkin, H., Bratman, G. N., Breslow, S. J., Cochran, B., Kahn, P. H., Jr., Lawler, J. J., & Wood, S. A. (2017). Nature contact and human health: A research agenda. Environmental Health Perspectives, 125(7), 075001. https://doi.org/10.1289/EHP1663

Kondo, M. C., Oyekanmi, K. O., Gibson, A., South, E. C., Bocarro, J., & Hipp, J. A. (2020). Nature prescriptions for health: A review of evidence and research opportunities. International Journal of Environmental Research and Public Health, 17(12), 4213. https://doi.org/10.3390/ijerph17124213

Nature Mental Health Editors. (2025). Climate change and the most vulnerable populations. Nature Mental Health. https://doi.org/10.1038/s44220-025-00570-9

Park Rx America. (2025). About Park Rx America. https://parkrxamerica.org/

Hinckson, E., Reis, R., Romanello, M., et al. (2026). Benefit of physical activity initiatives for climate change mitigation and adaptation. Nature Health, 1, 300–315. https://doi.org/10.1038/s44360-026-00057-6

Rashid, A., et al. (2026). Nature as medicine: A One Health approach to global health challenges. International Journal of Environmental Medicine, 1(1), 2. https://doi.org/10.3390/ijem1010002

Song, D., Kim, S., Park, M., et al. (2025). Thermal conditions modulate urban forest therapy outcomes: A meta-analytic review. Scientific Reports, 15, 39222. https://doi.org/10.1038/s41598-025-24331-x

White, M. P., Alcock, I., Grellier, J., Wheeler, B. W., Hartig, T., Warber, S. L., Bone, A., Depledge, M. H., & Fleming, L. E. (2019). Spending at least 120 minutes a week in nature is associated with good health and well-being. Scientific Reports, 9(1), 7730. https://doi.org/10.1038/s41598-019-44097-3

Wilson, E. O. (1984). Biophilia. Harvard University Press. https://www.hup.harvard.edu/catalog.php?isbn=9780674074422

# Afterword

Your choice to read **Get Out!** demonstrates a significant act because you chose to deliberately connect with nature, which society ignores in this digital era. That decision matters. The change represents a *deep, proactive choice* that leads to personal well-being by drawing from both scientific evidence and enduring wisdom.

The book demonstrates how contact with nature, through exposure to sunlight, the scent of pine after rain, and the sound of rustling leaves, produces *quantifiable improvements* in mood, focus, sleep quality, immunity, and mental clarity. The research findings that support these benefits originate from peer-reviewed studies and clinical investigations that you can now use to enhance your daily life. None of the studies represent the merchandising efforts often seen in TV ads that tout "clinical studies" frequently run by the manufacturers themselves.

Your commitment to reading this book suggests your interest in exploring *evidence-based wellness strategies developed by professionals.* Nothing that isn't substantiated by valid, professional research has been included, and we have been diligent not to include things deemed "hacks." *Question anything that is called a hack for your health.*

There is effort, there is knowledge, there is exploration, and there is beneficial curiosity. The importance of making well-informed decisions should be recognized in today's overwhelming landscape of self-help content. The decisions you make benefit everyone you encounter in your life. Your emotional growth into a centered, resilient version positively affects all those in your life, including family members, friends, coworkers, and members of your broader community.

Review the topics discussed, as they will reveal alternative paths forward and assist you in your quest for knowledge. Developing a relationship with nature is a lifelong journey, **not a one-time fix**. The information in this book should serve as your starting point while you explore beyond it. Your ongoing practice of walking, sitting, breathing, and being outdoors will persist.

The research findings in this book should inspire you to deepen your understanding through continuous learning. I have opened the door, or perhaps guided you to it, and now you can step through to expand your knowledge in every area that interests you and contributes to your health.

Thank you for choosing this path. Your commitment to health stands out because you approach self-improvement through thoughtful methods. You have started a journey that will create enduring changes that you can share with others. This book serves as a resource you will frequently visit, while its essential message reminds you that wellness exists right where your next breath of fresh air meets your body. By opting to read **Get Out!,** you've taken a *significant and powerful step*—you've made a *deliberate choice to re-establish a connection with the natural world*, which is often neglected in our hectic, digitally driven lives. That decision matters. It's more than a simple lifestyle shift; it's *a profound and proactive step toward personal well-being*, grounded in credible science and timeless wisdom.

# Bibliography

After each chapter there is a reference list for items utilized to write that chapter. This bibliography organizes the peer-reviewed research, books, and reports cited throughout **GET OUT!**, allowing readers, practitioners, and educators to locate source material quickly. References follow APA 7th edition format. Where available, DOI links and direct URLs are provided for access.

**Chapters 1 through 7** draw on research spanning several decades of environmental psychology, neuropsychology, and public health. **Chapters 8 through 10** incorporate research published through early 2026, reflecting the most current evidence base available at the time of writing.

American Society of Planning Officials. (1967, December). Vest pocket parks (Report No. 229). American Society of Planning Officials.

Antonelli M, Donelli D, Barbieri G, Valussi M, Maggini V, Firenzuoli F. Forest Volatile Organic Compounds and Their Effects on Human Health: A State-of-the-Art Review. Int J Environ Res Public Health. 2020 Sep 7;17(18):6506. doi: 10.3390/ijerph17186506. PMID: 32906736; PMCID: PMC7559006.

Alexander R, Nugent C, Nugent K. The Dust Bowl in the US: An Analysis Based on Current Environmental and Clinical Studies. Am J Med Sci. 2018 Aug;356(2):90-96. doi: 10.1016/j.amjms.2018.03.015. Epub 2018 Mar 26. PMID: 30219167.

Alvarsson, J. J., Wiens, S., & Nilsson, M. E. (2010). Stress recovery during exposure to nature sound and environmental noise. International Journal of Environmental Research and Public Health, 7(3), 1036–1046. https://doi.org/10.3390/ijerph7031036

Arent, S., Landers, D., & Etnier, J. (2000). The effects of exercise on mood in older adults: A meta-analytic review. Journal of Aging and Physical Activity, 8(4), 407–430. https://doi.org/10.1123/japa.8.4.407

Barton, J., & Pretty, J. (2010). What is the best dose of nature and green exercise for improving mental health? A multi-study analysis. Environmental Science & Technology, 44(10), 3947–3955. https://doi.org/10.1021/es903183r

BC Parks Foundation. (2025). PaRx: A nature prescription program. https://www.bcparksfoundation.ca/parx/

Bear, I. J., & Thomas, R. G. (1964). Nature of argillaceous odor. Nature, 201(4923), 993–995. https://www.nature.com/articles/201993a0

Bellón D, Rodriguez-Ayllon M, Solis-Urra P, Fernandez-Gamez B, Olvera-Rojas M, Coca-Pulido A, Toval A, Martín-Fuentes I, Bakker EA, Sclafani A, Fernández-Ortega J, Cabanas-Sánchez V, Mora-Gonzalez J, Gómez-Río M, Lubans DR, Ortega FB, Esteban-Cornejo I. Associations between muscular strength and mental health in cognitively normal older adults: a cross-sectional study from the AGUEDA trial. Int J Clin Health Psychol. 2024 Apr-Jun;24(2):100450. doi: 10.1016/j.ijchp.2024.100450. Epub 2024 Mar 19. PMID: 38525016; PMCID: PMC10960140

Berman, M. G., Jonides, J., & Kaplan, S. (2008). The cognitive benefits of interacting with nature. Psychological Science, 19(12), 1207–1212. https://doi.org/10.1111/j.1467-9280.2008.02225.x

Bielinis, E., et al. (2021). The effects of viewing a winter forest landscape on the psychological relaxation of young Finnish adults: A pilot study. PLOS ONE. https://doi.org/10.1371/journal.pone.0258856

Bratman, G. N., Anderson, C. B., Berman, M. G., et al. (2019). Nature and mental health: An ecosystem service perspective. Science Advances, 5(7), eaax0903. https://doi.org/10.1126/sciadv.aax0903

Bratman, G. N., Hamilton, J. P., Hahn, K. S., Daily, G. C., & Gross, J. J. (2015). Nature experience reduces rumination and subgenual prefrontal cortex activation. Proceedings of the National Academy of Sciences, 112(28), 8567–8572. https://doi.org/10.1073/pnas.1510459112

Browning, M. H. E. M., et al. (2020). Can simulated nature support mental health? Comparing short, single doses of 360-degree nature videos in virtual reality with the outdoors. Frontiers in Psychology, 11, 567200. https://doi.org/10.3389/fpsyg.2020.567200

Cacioppo, J. T., & Patrick, W. (2008). Loneliness: Human nature and the need for social connection. W.W. Norton & Company.

Cain, D., et al. (2025). Cold-water immersion: Systematic review of physiological and psychological effects. PLOS ONE. https://journals.plos.org/plosone/article?id=10.1371/journal.pone.0292321

Carlson, C. J., Mitchell, D., Gibb, R., et al. (2025). Health losses attributed to anthropogenic climate change. Nature Climate Change, 15, 1052–1055. https://doi.org/10.1038/s41558-025-02399-7

Center for American Progress. (2020). The nature gap: Confronting racial and economic disparities in the destruction and protection of nature in America. https://www.americanprogress.org/article/the-nature-gap/

Chekroud, S. R., Gueorguieva, R., Zheutlin, A. B., Paulus, M., Krumholz, H. M., Krystal, J. H., & Chekroud, A. M. (2018). Association between physical exercise and mental health in 1.2 million individuals in the USA between 2011 and 2015. The Lancet Psychiatry, 5(9), 739–746. https://doi.org/10.1016/S2213-0366(18)30227-X

Christian H, Bauman A, Epping JN, Levine GN, McCormack G, Rhodes RE, Richards E, Rock M, Westgarth C. Encouraging Dog Walking for Health Promotion and Disease Prevention. Am J Lifestyle Med. 2016 Apr 17;12(3):233-243. doi: 10.1177/155982761664368 6. PMID: 30202393; PMCID: PMC6124971.

Cleveland Clinic. (2024, June 18). Everything you need to know about habit stacking for self-improvement. Cleveland Clinic Health Essentials. https://health.clevelandclinic.org/habit-stacking

Coventry, P., et al. (2021). Nature-based outdoor activities for mental and physical health: Systematic review and meta-analysis. SSM—Population Health, 16, 100934. https://doi.org/10.1016/j.s smph.2021.100934

Cracknell, D., White, M. P., Pahl, S., Nichols, W. J., & Depledge, M. H. (2016). Marine nature experience and its significance to well-being: A qualitative study. International Journal of Wellbeing, 6(1). https: //doi.org/10.5502/ijw.v6i1.497

Czeisler, C. A., & Gooley, J. J. (2007). Sleep and circadian rhythms in humans. Cold Spring Harbor Symposia on Quantitative Biology, 72, 579–597. https://doi.org/10.1101/sqb.2007.72.064

Dennis LK, Vanbeek MJ, Beane Freeman LE, Smith BJ, Dawson DV, Coughlin JA. Sunburns and risk of cutaneous melanoma: does age matter? A comprehensive meta-analysis. Ann Epidemiol. 2008 Aug;18(8):614-27. doi: 10.1016/j.annepidem.2008.04.006. PMID: 18652979; PMCID: PMC2873840.

Duberstein, Adam & King, Betz & Johnson, Amy. (2021). Pit Bulls and Prejudice. The Humanistic Psychologist. 51. 183-188. 10.1037/hum0000259.

Epel, E., et al. (2025). Effects of a novel psychosocial climate resilience course on climate distress, self-efficacy, and mental health in young adults. Sustainability, 17, 3139. https://doi.org/10.3390/su17073139

Epley, N., & Schroeder, J. (2014). Mistakenly seeking solitude. Journal of Experimental Psychology: General, 143(5), 1980–1999. https://doi.org/10.1037/a0037323

Evans, G. W., & Lepore, S. J. (1993). Nonauditory effects of noise on children: A critical review. Children's Environments, 10(1), 31–51. https://www.jstor.org/stable/41514773

Fan, W., Oh, T. G., Wang, H. J., Crossley, L., He, M., Robbins, H., Koopari, C., Dai, Y., Truitt, M. L., Liddle, C., Yu, R. T., Atkins, A. R., Downes, M., & Evans, R. M. (2025). Estrogen-related receptors regulate innate and adaptive muscle mitochondrial energetics through cooperative and distinct actions. Proceedings of the National Academy of Sciences, 122(20), e2426179122. https://doi.org/10.1073/pnas.2426179122

Fascitelli, Jack. (2019). Robert Moses and the Real Estate City: A Reexamination of the Legacy of New York's Master Builder [Documents]. Trinity Student Scholarship. Trinity College Digital Repository. https://jstor.org/stable/community.34031347

Ferrario, M., Piccolo, E., Lanzini, M., De Mita, A. C., & Giannattasio, C. (2021). Physiological effects of natural sound on surgical recovery. Pain Medicine, 22(11), 2517–2526. https://doi.org/10.1093/pm/pnab142

Finley AJ, Schaefer SM. Affective Neuroscience of Loneliness: Potential Mechanisms underlying the Association between Perceived Social Isolation, Health, and Well-Being. J Psychiatr Brain Sci. 2022;7(6):e220011. doi: 10.20900/jpbs.20220011. Epub 2022 Dec 26. PMID: 36778655; PMCID: PMC9910279.

Fontana, K. (2026, March 13). Campus health now offering nature prescriptions. NC State Global One Health Academy. https://provost.ncsu.edu/global-one-health-academy/2026/03/13/campus-health-now-offering-nature-prescriptions/

Fournier, M., et al. (2017). Effects of a text-messaging intervention on physical activity: A meta-analysis. Behavioral Medicine, 43(4), 263–274. https://doi.org/10.1080/08964289.2016.1222347

Frumkin, H., Bratman, G. N., Breslow, S. J., Cochran, B., Kahn, P. H., Jr., Lawler, J. J., & Wood, S. A. (2017). Nature contact and human health: A research agenda. Environmental Health Perspectives, 125(7), 075001. https://doi.org/10.1289/EHP1663

Gardner, B., Rebar, A. L., & Lally, P. (2020). A matter of habit: Recognizing the multiple roles of habit in health behaviour. British Journal of General Practice, 70(699), 514–515. https://doi.org/10.3399/bjgp20X712597

Gidlow, C. J., Jones, M. V., Hurst, G., Masterson, D., Clark-Carter, D., Tarvainen, M. P., Smith, G., & Nieuwenhuijsen, M. (2016). Where to find nature's lead? A systematic review and meta-analysis. British Journal of Sports Medicine, 50(18), 1176–1183. https://doi.org/10.1136/bjsports-2015-095687

Gollwitzer, P. M. (1999). Implementation intentions: Strong effects of simple plans. American Psychologist, 54(7), 493–503. https://doi.org/10.1037/0003-066X.54.7.493

Hammoud, R., Tognin, S., Burgess, L., Bergou, N., Smythe, M., Gibbons, J., Davidson, N., Afifi, A., Bakolis, I., & Bhome, R. (2022). Smartphone-based ecological momentary assessment reveals mental health benefits of birdlife. Scientific Reports, 12, 17589. https://doi.org/10.1038/s41598-022-20207-6

Harvey, A. G., & Gumport, N. B. (2022). Applying the science of habit formation to evidence-based psychological treatments for mental illness. Perspectives on Psychological Science, 17(2), 572–589. https://doi.org/10.1177/1745691621995752

Hasan MK. Digital multitasking and hyperactivity: unveiling the hidden costs to brain health. Ann Med Surg (Lond). 2024 Sep 18;86(11):6371-6373. doi: 10.1097/MS9.0000000000002576 . PMID: 39525791; PMCID: PMC11543232.

Hansen MM, Jones R, Tocchini K. Shinrin-Yoku (Forest Bathing) and Nature Therapy: A State-of-the-Art Review. Int J Environ Res Public Health. 2017 Jul 28;14(8):851. doi: 10.3390/ijerph14080851. PMID: 28788101; PMCID: PMC5580555.

Hoffmann C, Weigert C. Skeletal Muscle as an Endocrine Organ: The Role of Myokines in Exercise Adaptations. Cold Spring Harb Perspect Med. 2017 Nov 1;7(11):a029793. doi: 10.1101/cshperspect.a029793. PMID: 28389517; PMCID: PMC5666622

Holick, M. F. (2004). Vitamin D: Importance in the prevention of cancers, type 1 diabetes, heart disease, and osteoporosis. American Journal of Clinical Nutrition, 79(3), 362–371. https://doi.org/10.1093/ajcn/79.3.362

Holick, M. F. (2007). Vitamin D deficiency. New England Journal of Medicine, 357(3), 266–281. https://doi.org/10.1056/NEJMra070553

Holt-Lunstad, J., Smith, T. B., Baker, M., Harris, T., & Stephenson, D. (2015). Loneliness and social isolation as risk factors for mortality: A meta-analytic review. Perspectives on Psychological Science, 10(2), 227–237. https://doi.org/10.1177/1745691614568352

Hui, X., et al. (2025). Virtual nature, real relief: How exposure to virtual natural environments reduces anxiety, stress, and depression in healthy adults. npj Digital Medicine, 8, 679. https://doi.org/10.1038/s41746-025-02057-4

Hunter, M. R., Gillespie, B. W., & Chen, S. Y. P. (2019). Urban nature experiences reduce stress in the context of daily life based on salivary biomarkers. Frontiers in Psychology, 10, 722. https://doi.org/10.3389/fpsyg.2019.00722

Ichihara Y, Mori H, Kamada M, Matsuura T, Sairyo K, Hyodo M, Tsutsumi R, Sakaue H, Aihara KI, Funaki M, Kuroda A, Matsuhisa M. Effects of high-intensity interval walking training on muscle strength, walking ability, and health-related quality of life in people with diabetes accompanied by lower extremity weakness: A randomized controlled trial. J Diabetes Investig. 2025 Apr;16(4):646-655. doi: 10.1111/jdi.14399. Epub 2025 Jan 7. PMID: 39776311; PMCID: PMC11970289.

Iglesias P. Muscle in Endocrinology: From Skeletal Muscle Hormone Regulation to Myokine Secretion and Its Implications in Endocrine-Metabolic Diseases. J Clin Med. 2025 Jun 25;14(13):4490. doi: 10.3390/jcm14134490. PMID: 40648864; PMCID: PMC12249830

Inglis-Arkell, E. (2014, October 8). The problem with the famously godawful executive monkey study. Gizmodo. https://gizmodo.com/the-problem-with-the-famously-godawful-executive-monkey-1643699082

Jiayu He, Yuanning Guo, Jiamin Chen, Jinhua Xu, Xiaohua Zhu. Exploring the correlation between UVB sensitivity and SLE activity: Insights into UVB-driven pathogenesis in lupus erythematosus, Journal of Autoimmunity, Volume 153, 2025, 103393, ISSN

0896-8411, https://doi.org/10.1016/j.jaut.2025.103393. (https://www.sciencedirect.com/science/article/pii/S0896841125000381).

Kaplan, R., & Kaplan, S. (1989). The experience of nature: A psychological perspective. Cambridge University Press.

Kaplan, S. (1995). The restorative benefits of nature: Toward an integrative framework. Journal of Environmental Psychology, 15(3), 169–182. https://doi.org/10.1016/0272-4944(95)90001-2

Keltner, D. (2023). Awe: The new science of everyday wonder and how it can transform your life. Penguin Press.

Keltner, D., & Haidt, J. (2003). Approaching awe, a moral, spiritual, and aesthetic emotion. Cognition and Emotion, 17(2), 297–314. https://doi.org/10.1080/02699930302297

Kim A, Chong BF. Photosensitivity in cutaneous lupus erythematosus. Photodermatol Photoimmunol Photomed. 2013 Feb;29(1):4-11. doi: 10.1111/phpp.12018. PMID: 23281691; PMCID: PMC3539182.

Klein, D. C. (2016). The pineal gland and melatonin. In J. L. Jameson & L. J. De Groot (Eds.), Endocrinology: Adult and pediatric (7th ed., pp. 312–322). W.B. Saunders. https://doi.org/10.1016/B978-0-323-18907-1.00019-6

Knechtle, B., et al. (2020). Cold water swimming—benefits and risks: A narrative review. International Journal of Environmental Research and Public Health, 17(23), 8984. https://www.mdpi.com/1660-4601/17/23/8984

Kondo, M. C., Fluehr, J. M., McKeon, T., & Branas, C. C. (2018). Urban green space and its impact on human health. International Journal of Environmental Research and Public Health, 15(3), 445. https://doi.org/10.3390/ijerph15030445

Kondo, M. C., Oyekanmi, K. O., Gibson, A., South, E. C., Bocarro, J., & Hipp, J. A. (2020). Nature prescriptions for health: A review of evidence and research opportunities. International Journal of Environmental Research and Public Health, 17(12), 4213. https://doi.org/10.3390/ijerph17124213

Krause, B. (2012). The great animal orchestra: Finding the origins of music in the world's wild places. Little, Brown and Company.

Kuo, F. E., & Faber Taylor, A. (2004). A potential natural treatment for attention-deficit/hyperactivity disorder: Evidence from a national study. American Journal of Public Health, 94(9), 1580–1586. https://doi.org/10.2105/AJPH.94.9.1580

Lally, P., van Jaarsveld, C. H. M., Potts, H. W. W., & Wardle, J. (2010). How are habits formed: Modeling habit formation in the real world. European Journal of Social Psychology, 40(6), 998–1009. https://doi.org/10.1002/ejsp.674

Lambert, G. W., Reid, C., Kaye, D. M., Jennings, G. L., & Esler, M. D. (2002). Effect of sunlight and season on serotonin turnover in the brain. The Lancet, 360(9348), 1840–1842. https://doi.org/10.1016/S0140-6736(02)11737-5

Laszlo, H. E., McRobie, E. S., Stansfeld, S. A., & Hansell, A. L. (2012). Residential road traffic noise and mental health: An urban perspective. Noise & Health, 14(58), 99–107. https://doi.org/10.4103/1463-1741.95138

Li, Q. (2010). Effect of forest bathing trips on human immune function. Environmental Health and Preventive Medicine, 15(1), 9–17. https://doi.org/10.1007/s12199-008-0068-3

Mai Charlotte Krogh Severinsen, Bente Klarlund Pedersen. Muscle–Organ Crosstalk: The Emerging Roles of Myokines, Endocrine Reviews, Volume 41, Issue 4, August 2020, Pages 594–609, https://doi.org/10.1210/endrev/bnaa016

Marselle, M. R., Martens, D., Dallimer, M., & Irvine, K. N. (2020). Review of the mental health and well-being benefits of biodiversity.

In M. R. Marselle et al. (Eds.), Biodiversity and health in the face of climate change. Springer, Cham. https://doi.org/10.1007/978-3-030-02318-8_10

Martland, R., Mondelli, V., Gaughran, F., & Stubbs, B. (2020). Can high-intensity interval training improve physical and mental health outcomes? A meta-review of 33 systematic reviews. Journal of Sports Sciences, 38(4), 430–469. https://doi.org/10.1080/02640414.2019.1706829

Matsunaga, K., et al. (2011). Aromatic effects of a Japanese forest on mood and stress in female university students. International Journal of Environmental Research and Public Health, 8(9), 3532–3542. https://www.mdpi.com/1660-4601/8/9/3532

Medvedev, O., Shepherd, D., & Hautus, M. J. (2015). The restorative potential of soundscapes: A physiological investigation. Applied Acoustics, 96, 20–26. https://doi.org/10.1016/j.apacoust.2015.03.004

Melrose S. Seasonal Affective Disorder: An Overview of Assessment and Treatment Approaches. Depress Res Treat. 2015;2015:178564. doi: 10.1155/2015/178564. Epub 2015 Nov 25. PMID: 26688752; PMCID: PMC4673349.

Milkman, K. L. (2021). How to change: The science of getting from where you are to where you want to be. Portfolio/Penguin.

Mitchell, R., & Popham, F. (2008). Effect of exposure to natural environment on health inequalities: An observational population study. The Lancet, 372(9650), 1655–1660. https://doi.org/10.1016/S0140-6736(08)61689-X

Morita, E., Fukuda, S., Nagano, J., Hamajima, N., Yamamoto, H., Iwai, Y., Nakashima, T., Ohira, H., & Shirakawa, T. (2007). Psychological effects of forest environments on healthy adults. Public Health, 121(1), 54–63. https://doi.org/10.1016/j.puhe.2006.05.024

Nature Mental Health Editors. (2025). Climate change and the most vulnerable populations. Nature Mental Health. https://doi.org/10.1038/s44220-025-00570-9

Naumann RK, Ondracek JM, Reiter S, Shein-Idelson M, Tosches MA, Yamawaki TM, Laurent G. The reptilian brain. Curr Biol. 2015 Apr 20;25(8):R317-21. doi: 10.1016/j.cub.2015.02.049. PMID: 25898097; PMCID: PMC4406946.

Neff, E.P. Stop and smell the geosmin. Lab Anim 47, 270 (2018). https://doi.org/10.1038/s41684-018-0161-1

Nguyen CTO, Acosta ML, Di Angelantonio S, Salt TE. Editorial: Seeing Beyond the Eye: The Brain Connection. Front Neurosci. 2021 Jun 29;15:719717. doi: 10.3389/fnins.2021.719717. PMID: 34267626; PMCID: PMC8276094.

Nichols, W. J. (2014). Blue mind: The surprising science that shows how being near, in, on, or under water can make you happier, healthier, more connected, and better at what you do. Little, Brown and Company

Ogura A, Izawa KP, Tawa H, Kureha F, Wada M, Harada N, Ikeda Y, Kimura K, Kondo N, Kanai M, Kubo I, Yoshikawa R, Matsuda Y. Older phase 2 cardiac rehabilitation patients engaged in gardening maintained physical function during the COVID-19 pandemic. Heart Vessels. 2022 Jan;37(1):77-82. doi: 10.1007/s00380-021-01892-1. Epub 2021 Jun 21. PMID: 34152441; PMCID: PMC8215626.

Pail, G., Huf, W., Pjrek, E., Winkler, D., Willeit, M., Praschak-Rieder, N., & Kasper, S. (2011). Bright-light therapy in the treatment of mood disorders. Neuropsychobiology, 64(3), 152–162. https://doi.org/10.1159/000328950

Park, B. J., Tsunetsugu, Y., Kasetani, T., Kagawa, T., & Miyazaki, Y. (2010). The physiological effects of Shinrin-yoku: Evidence from field experiments in 24 forests across Japan. Environmental Health and

Preventive Medicine, 15(1), 18–26. https://doi.org/10.1007/s12199-009-0086-9

Park Rx America. (2025). About Park Rx America. https://parkrxamerica.org/

Peen, J., Schoevers, R. A., Beekman, A. T., & Dekker, J. (2010). The current status of urban-rural differences in psychiatric disorders. Acta Psychiatrica Scandinavica, 121(2), 84–93. https://doi.org/10.1111/j.1600-0447.2009.01438.x

Pogash, C. (2026, April 18). This Bay Area 80-year-old sets marathon records. Here's what her story says about aging. San Francisco Chronicle. https://www.sfchronicle.com/health/aging-longevity/article/patty-hung-marathon-runner-22183907.php

Pratesi A, Tarantini F, Di Bari M. Skeletal muscle: an endocrine organ. Clin Cases Miner Bone Metab. 2013 Jan;10(1):11-4. doi: 10.11138/ccmbm/2013.10.1.011. PMID: 23858303; PMCID: PMC3710002

Pretty, J., Peacock, J., Sellens, M., & Griffin, M. (2005). The mental and physical health outcomes of green exercise. International Journal of Environmental Health Research, 15(5), 319–337 https://doi.org/10.1080/09603120500155963

Rashid, A., et al. (2026). Nature as medicine: A One Health approach to global health challenges. International Journal of Environmental Medicine, 1(1), 2. https://doi.org/10.3390/ijem1010002

Richardson, M., Cormack, A., McRobert, L., & Underhill, R. (2016). 30 days wild: Development and evaluation of a large-scale nature engagement campaign to improve well-being. PLOS ONE, 11(2), e0149777. https://doi.org/10.1371/journal.pone.0149777

Rigolon, A., Browning, M., McAnirlin, O., & Yoon, H. V. (2021). Green space and health equity: A systematic review. International

Journal of Environmental Research and Public Health, 18(5), 2563. https://doi.org/10.3390/ijerph18052563

Roecklein, K. A., & Rohan, K. J. (2005). Seasonal affective disorder: An overview and update. Psychiatry, 2(1), 20–26. https://pubmed.ncbi.nlm.nih.gov/23878527/

Schubert, D. (2019). Jane Jacobs, cities, urban planning, ethics and value systems. Cities, 91, 4-9. https://doi.org/10.1016/j.cities.2018.05.001

Shaffer, J. A., Bhatt, D. L., & Bhatt, N. (2022). Outdoor time and mental health: Large-scale analysis of daylight exposure and depression risk. JAMA Psychiatry, 79(4), 330–339. https://doi.org/10.1001/jamapsychiatry.2021.4359

Shampo MA, Kyle RA, Steensma DP. Edward L. Trudeau--founder of a sanatorium for treatment of tuberculosis. Mayo Clin Proc. 2010 Jul;85(7):e48. doi: 10.4065/mcp.2010.0379. PMID: 20592164; PMCID: PMC2894729.

Sinczuk, M., et al. (2011). Effects of winter swimming on haematological parameters. Biochemia Medica. https://doi.org/10.11613/BM.2011.035

Soga, M., & Gaston, K. J. (2025). Health benefits of viewing nature through windows: A meta-analysis. BioScience, 75(8), 628–640. https://doi.org/10.1093/biosci/biaf059

Soga, M., Gaston, K. J., & Yamaura, Y. (2017). Gardening is beneficial for health: A meta-analysis. Preventive Medicine Reports, 5, 92–99. https://doi.org/10.1016/j.pmedr.2016.11.007

Soga, M., et al. (2025). A systematic review and meta-analysis on the effect of nature exposure dose on adults with mental illness. PMC11851813. https://pmc.ncbi.nlm.nih.gov/articles/PMC11851813/

Song, D., Kim, S., Park, M., et al. (2025). Thermal conditions modulate urban forest therapy outcomes: A meta-analytic review. Scientific Reports, 15, 39222. https://doi.org/10.1038/s41598-025-24331-x

South, E. C., Hohl, B. C., Kondo, M. C., MacDonald, J. M., & Branas, C. C. (2018). Effect of greening vacant land on mental health of community-dwelling adults: A cluster randomized trial. JAMA Network Open, 1(3), e180298. https://doi.org/10.1001/jamanetw orkopen. 2018.0298

Suess, C., & Maddock, J. (2025). Understanding the influence of window views, plantscapes, and green decor in virtual reality hospital rooms on simulated acute-care patients' stress recovery and relaxation responses. HERD, 18(3), 165–183. https://doi.org/10.1177/19375 867251344626

Sullivan, W. C., Kuo, F. E., & DePooter, S. F. (2004). The fruit of urban nature: Vital neighborhood spaces. Environment and Behavior, 36(5), 678–700. https://doi.org/10.1177/0193841X04264945

Sutin AR, Luchetti M, Aschwanden D, Lee JH, Sesker AA, Stephan Y, Terracciano A. Sense of purpose in life and concurrent loneliness and risk of incident loneliness: An individual-participant meta-analysis of 135,227 individuals from 36 cohorts. J Affect Disord. 2022 Jul 15;309:211-220. doi: 10.1016/j.jad.2022.04.084. Epub 2022 Apr 26. PMID: 35483500; PMCID: PMC9133197.

Tahkamo, L., Partonen, T., & Pesonen, A. K. (2019). Systematic review of light exposure impact on human circadian rhythm. Chronobiology International, 36(2), 151–170. https://doi.org/10.1 080/07420528.2018.1527773

Tanner, R. (2026, April 24). London Marathon: Hundreds of over-70s are running. This is what motivates them. The Athletic. https://www.nytimes.com/athletic/7141362/2026/04/24/lond on-marathon-2026-senior-runners-ever-presents/

Tao, J., Li, X., Stenfors, C. U. D., Rumble, A., & Nilsson, M. E. (2021). Effects of birdsong on urban residents' restoration. Environmental Research, 195, 110299. https://doi.org/10.1016/j.envres.2020.110299

Thompson Coon, J., Boddy, K., Stein, K., Whear, R., Barton, J., & Depledge, M. H. (2011). Does participating in physical activity in outdoor natural environments have a greater effect on physical and mental well-being than indoors? Environmental Science & Technology, 45(5), 1761–1772. https://doi.org/10.1021/es102947t

Tsunetsugu, Y., Park, B. J., & Miyazaki, Y. (2010). Trends in research related to Shinrin-yoku in Japan. Environmental Health and Preventive Medicine, 15(1), 27–37. https://doi.org/10.1007/s12199-009-0091-z

Twenge, J. M. (2017). iGen: Why today's super-connected kids are growing up less rebellious, more tolerant, less happy—and completely unprepared for adulthood. Atria Books.

Tyrvainen, L., et al. (2014). The influence of urban green environments on stress relief measures: A field experiment. Journal of Environmental Psychology, 38, 1–9. https://doi.org/10.1016/j.jenvp.2013.12.005

Uebi, T., et al. (2021). Geosmin triggers a pleasant neural response in humans. Frontiers in Neuroscience, 15. https://doi.org/10.3389/fnins.2021.674394

Ulrich, R. S. (1984). View through a window may influence recovery from surgery. Science, 224(4647), 420–421. https://doi.org/10.1126/science.6143402

Ulrich, R. S., Simons, R. F., Losito, B. D., Fiorito, E., Miles, M. A., & Zelson, M. (1991). Stress recovery during exposure to natural and urban environments. Journal of Environmental Psychology, 11(3), 201–230. https://doi.org/10.1016/S0272-4944(05)80184-7

Umucu, E., et al. (2025). Health inequities among persons with disabilities: A global scoping review. Frontiers in Public Health, 13, 1538519. https://doi.org/10.3389/fpubh.2025.1538519

U.S. Department of Health and Human Services. (2023). Our epidemic of loneliness and isolation: The U.S. Surgeon General's advisory on the healing effects of social connection and community. Office of the Surgeon General. https://www.hhs.gov/sites/default/files/surgeon-general-social-connection-advisory.pdf

Vo, D., et al. (2026). The impact of virtual reality-based forest therapy in psychiatric inpatient care: A pilot study. Advances in Mental Health. https://doi.org/10.1080/18387357.2026.2615679

Walser, L. (2016, April 14). A tale of two planners: Jane Jacobs vs. Robert Moses. Saving Places. https://savingplaces.org/stories/a-tale-of-two-planners-jane-jacobs-and-robert-moses

Wheeler, B. W., White, M., Stahl-Timmins, W., & Depledge, M. H. (2012). Does living by the coast improve health and well-being? Health & Place, 18(5), 1198–1201. https://doi.org/10.1016/j.healthplace.2012.06.015

White, M. P., Alcock, I., Grellier, J., Wheeler, B. W., Hartig, T., Warber, S. L., Bone, A., Depledge, M. H., & Fleming, L. E. (2019). Spending at least 120 minutes a week in nature is associated with good health and well-being. Scientific Reports, 9(1), 7730. https://doi.org/10.1038/s41598-019-44097-3

White, M. P., Elliott, L. R., Gascon, M., Roberts, B., & Fleming, L. E. (2020). Blue space, health and well-being: A narrative overview and synthesis of potential benefits. Environmental Research, 191. https://doi.org/10.1016/j.envres.2020.110169

White, M. P., et al. (2018). A prescription for 'nature'—the potential of using virtual nature in therapeutics. Neuropsychiatric Disease and Treatment, 14, 3001–3013. https://doi.org/10.2147/NDT.S179038

Wilson, E. O. (1984). Biophilia. Harvard University Press. https://www.hup.harvard.edu/catalog.php?isbn=9780674074422

Wolff, M., & Wehr, T. A. (2023). Green exercise and depression: A meta-analysis of randomized controlled trials. Environmental Health Perspectives, 131(3), 037001. https://doi.org/10.1289/EHP11003

Wood, W. (2026, January). Wendy Wood helps people apply the science of habits in everyday life. Monitor on Psychology, 57(1). https://www.apa.org/monitor/2026/01-02/wendy-wood-habits-behavior-change

Wood, W., & Neal, D. T. (2016). Healthy through habit: Interventions for initiating and maintaining health behavior change. Behavioral Science & Policy, 2(1), 71–83. https://doi.org/10.1353/bsp.2016.0008

Yau, K. K. Y., & Loke, A. Y. (2021). Effects of forest bathing on pre-hypertensive and hypertensive adults: A review of the literature. Environmental Health and Preventive Medicine, 26(1), 25. https://doi.org/10.1186/s12199-021-00941-3

Ye, X., et al. (2024). Reduction in socioeconomic inequalities in self-reported mental health conditions with increasing greenspace exposure. PMC11151689. https://pmc.ncbi.nlm.nih.gov/articles/PMC11151689/

Zahrt, O. H., & Crum, A. J. (2017). Perceived physical activity and mortality: Evidence from three nationally representative U.S. samples. Health Psychology, 36(11), 1017–1025. https://doi.org/10.1037/hea0000531

Zhang, J. W., Howell, R. T., & Iyer, R. (2014). Engagement with natural beauty moderates the positive relation between connectedness with nature and psychological well-being. Journal of Environmental Psychology, 38, 55–63. https://doi.org/10.1016/j.jenvp.2013.12.013

Zhou, X., Rosini, J. M., & Bhatt, D. L. (2023). Long-term traffic noise exposure and risk of depression: A population-based study of two million adults. The Lancet Regional Health—Americas, 18, 100406. https://doi.org/10.1016/j.lana.2022.100406

# About the Author

Dr. Patricia A. Farrell is a licensed psychologist, published author of multiple self-help books and videos, former WebMD psychologist expert/consultant, medical consultant for Social Security Disability Determinations, Alzheimer's psychiatric researcher at Mt. Sinai Medical Center (NYC), an educator who has taught at the college, graduate, and postgraduate levels, and top health writer for *Medium.com* publications and her *Patreon blog, "Dr. Farrell Unplugged."* A flash fiction writer, she has had her stories published over 40 times in various magazines.

Her influence extends to the pharmaceutical and marketing industries, where she serves as a consultant and has appeared on major TV news programs in the US and abroad. In addition, Dr. Farrell provides continuing education modules for mental healthcare professionals and has contributed to USMLE medical school prep courses. She shares her knowledge through her YouTube channel and her daily contributions to **Bluesky** (@carpenter22,bsky.social). Dr. Farrell's achievements are recognized in *Who's Who in the World, Who's Who in America,* and *Who's Who in American Women.*

A member of the American Psychological Association and the SAG-AFTRA union, Dr. Farrell is a former board member of the NJ

Board of Psychological Examiners, a former psychiatry preceptor at UMDNJ, and a former board of directors member of Bergen Pines Hospital (now Bergen Regional Hospital).

**Books by Patricia A. Farrell, Ph.D.**

When You Can't Pour From an Empty Glass: CBT Skills for Exhausted Caregivers.

The Little Book on Learning Big Critical Thinking Skills

The Smart Kids' Survival Guide: Making Good Choices in a Confusing World

How to Be Your Own Therapist

It's Not All in Your Head: Anxiety, Depression, Mood Swings and Multiple Sclerosis

Unfiltered: Beneath the noise of our thoughts lies the true narrative of our minds

Unfiltered Again: A behind-the-scenes look at healthcare, medicine and mental health

Unfiltered Redux: Exploring uncharted depths of mind where masks fall and wisdom emerges

A Social Security Disability Psychological Claims Handbook: A simple guide to understanding your SSD claim for psychological impairments and unraveling the maze of decision-making

A Social Security Disability Psychological Claims Guidebook for Children's Benefits

The Disability Accessible US Parks in All 50 States: A Comprehensive Guide

Birding in the US NOW!: A birding guide for individuals with disabilities

# A Special Request

If this book has touched your heart, sparked your curiosity, or simply entertained you along the way, I'd be incredibly grateful if you could take a moment to share your thoughts with a review on Amazon or wherever you discovered this book. Your words not only help other readers find books they'll love, but they also mean the world to authors like me who pour their hearts into every page. Thank you for being part of this journey, and for helping stories find their way to the readers who need them most.

*Author Page on Amazon: https://tinyurl.com/4ewdunb8*

# Reviews

**Dr. Allan Frances**, renowned psychiatrist, currently Professor and Chairman Emeritus of the Department of Psychiatry and Behavioral Sciences at *Duke University School of Medicine.*

*"Nature is a great healer of psychiatric problems—bringing joy, inspiring hope, providing meaning, reversing demoralization. And Nature is everywhere if only we pay attention to it. This book combines inspiration, wisdom, and good practical advice."*

**Gil Bashe,** Chair Globalhealth and Purpose, FINN Partners and Editor-in-Chief, Medika Life

*"Get Out" is a brilliant, expansive work that gets us out of our heads. Dr. Patricia Farrell, a seasoned psychologist, knows we are flesh and blood, thoughts and feelings. Her wisdom helps readers recognize that emotional and physical healing calls for a multisensory life approach. "Get Out" is a perfect personal guide for life's earth, wind, and fire journey."*

www.ingramcontent.com/pod-product-compliance
Lightning Source LLC
LaVergne TN
LVHW090604110826
845146LV00001B/251

* 9 7 9 8 9 9 3 7 3 9 6 9 4 *